The ICU Therapeutics Handbook

Paul E. Marik

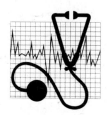

The ICU Therapeutics Handbook

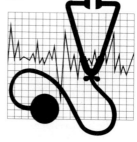

Paul Ellis Marik, MBBCh, FCP(SA),
FRCP(C), M.Med, BSc Hons (Pharmacology), DA

Assistant Professor of Medicine
University of Massachusetts Medical School
and
Director of the Medical Intensive Care Unit
Saint Vincent Hospital
Worcester, Massachusetts

with *38* illustrations

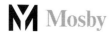 Mosby

St. Louis Baltimore Berlin Boston
Carlsbad Chicago London Madrid Naples
New York Philadelphia Portland Sydney Tokyo Toronto

Vice-President and Publisher: Anne S. Patterson
Senior Editor: Laurel Craven
Senior Developmental Editor: Sandra Clark Brown
Project Manager: Mark Spann
Senior Production Editor: Amy Adams Squire Strongheart
Designer: Judi Lang
Manufacturing Supervisor: Tony McAllister
Clipart images provided by Image Club Graphics, Inc.
@ 1-800-661-9410.

Copyright ©1996 by Mosby–Year Book, Inc.

Printed in the United States of America
Composition/lithography by V & M Graphics Incorporated
Printing/binding by R. R. Donnelley and Sons, Inc.

Mosby–Year Book, Inc.
11830 Westline Industrial Drive
St. Louis, MO 63146

Library of Congress Cataloging in Publication Data
Marik, Paul Ellis.
  The ICU therapeutics handbook / Paul Ellis Marik.
     p.   cm.
  Includes index.
  ISBN 0-8151-5698-7
  1. Critical care medicine—Handbooks, manuals, etc.   I. Title.
  [DNLM: 1. Intensive Care—methods—handbooks.   2. Critical
Illness—therapy—handbooks.   3. Intensive Care Units—organization
& administration—handbooks.   WX 39 M335i 1996]
  RC86.8.M385   1996
  616*.028—dc20
  DNLM/DLC
  for Library of Congress   95-51011
                                                                    CIP

96   97   98   99   00   /   9   8   7   6   5   4   3   2   1

To Kathryn and Emma,
for their love and understanding

Foreword

Most critical care physicians whom I know spend the 2 or 3 days before their turn in the ICU (be it 1 week or 1 month) with a sense of vague unease and mild dyspepsia, a state that I have decided is less attributable to the dread of acute illnesses than to the dread of dealing with the jumble of high-tech numbers, alarms, and machines that have now become a part of all ICUs. And if attending physicians feel this way, one can only imagine what goes through the mind of interns, residents, and fellows before their rotations.

I have found no good cure for this particular malaise, but Dr. Paul Marik, a seasoned critical care clinician, with this book, has given us the best hope so far for such a cure. It is a book that can be read cover to cover in one or two sittings and still manages to provide enough detail in the management of specific problems to be useful as a guide to be used every day in the ICU.

The book is organized into 66 chapters, each dealing with problems regularly encountered in the ICU. Since all of the chapters have been written by Dr. Marik, there is a consistency of style and philosophy sorely missing from other multiauthor books. Each chapter contains a wealth of information on diagnostic strategies, management options and recommendations, and nuggets of information, including relevant, but often difficult to track down, formulas and drug doses. Without pretending to be comprehensive, Dr. Marik manages quite well to cover nearly all of the diagnostic and management issues that one normally sees in the ICU. The book manages to convey a sense of having a wise clinician at one's side at all times.

This book has no references, a conscious decision made by the author to avoid distracting the reader as so many other textbooks do. Obviously, the conscientious reader will supplement his or her reading with more extensive reading in either one of the larger ICU textbooks or a standard internal medicine or surgery text; likewise, this book is not a substitute for careful library and journal study.

What this book does do so admirably is to make comprehensible to the reader the most daunting aspects of critical care medicine, in such a way that the reader is freed to concentrate on the problems and patients at hand. For anyone who practices regularly in the ICU, this is the *sine qua non* for good practice. One must be able to cut through the maze of extraneous "stuff" that has cluttered up the ICU to actually get to care for the patient. *The ICU Therapeutics Handbook* is of excellent help in pursuit of this goal.

I will ask my residents to read this book at least once or twice before beginning their ICU rotations and then have them keep it with them throughout their rotation. I am confident that these residents, fellows, and ICU attendants will find this book to be as useful as I have found it.

John A. Day, Jr., M.D.
Assistant Professor of Medicine
University of Massachusetts Medical School
Saint Vincent Hospital
Worcester, Massachusetts

Preface

The ICU Therapeutics Handbook is not a reference text but rather a "how to do it guide." This handbook was written to provide practical guidelines for clinicians involved in the daily care of ICU patients. Standardized diagnostic and therapeutic protocols are provided that incorporate up-to-date information. Critically ill ICU patients, however, have complex medical problems for which there is no simple approach. The optimal management of these patients requires close bedside observation, obsessive attention to detail, the integration of a large data base of knowledge, and good clinical judgment.

Acknowledgements

The following individuals are recognized for their contribution to this book: Navin Jain, M.D., for his editorial assistance and coauthorship of Chapters 47, 58, and 59; and John Day, M.D. and Wendy Lancey, R.N. for their invaluable advice; the medical residents at Saint Vincent Hospital who encouraged me to write this book; and my administrative assistant Mrs. Jackie Calcia.

Paul Ellis Marik

Contents

PART THREE
Metabolic and Endocrine Problems in the ICU

PART FOUR
The Gastrointestinal Tract

PART FIVE
Neurology

PART SIX
Infectious Diseases

PART SEVEN
Miscellaneous ICU Topics

PART EIGHT
In a Lighter Vein

PART ONE

THE RESPIRATORY SYSTEM

CHAPTER 1

Airway management

Endotracheal intubation

INDICATIONS FOR INTUBATION

- Acute or impending respiratory failure
- Upper airway obstruction
- Airway trauma
- Inhalational injury
- Upper airway bleeding
- Loss of airway reflexes and airway protection
    Central nervous system diseases
    Stupor and coma
    Massive upper GI bleeding
- Tracheobronchial suctioning
- Apnea
- Flail chest
- Management of increased intracranial pressure

ROUTE OF INTUBATION

Endotracheal intubation can be accomplished by either the orotracheal or nasotracheal route. Each has its specific advantages and disadvantages. In general, orotracheal intubation is preferred because it is rapid, more frequently successful, and allows a larger tube to be used. Blind nasotracheal intubation is, however, often preferred in the conscious patient because it affords greater patient comfort, is usually well tolerated, and does not require anesthesia. Furthermore, the tube is more stable, easier to secure, and mouth care is easier.

Patients who are nasally intubated are at a high risk of developing sinusitis. Almost all patients with a nasotracheal tube in situ will develop opacification of the paranasal sinuses within 3 days. Many of these patients will subsequently develop bacterial sinusitis. Therefore, if intubation for longer than 3 days is anticipated, patients should be intubated orally.

Contraindications to nasotracheal intubation include the following:

- Apnea
- A bleeding diathesis
- Nasal polyps

It has been taught that patients with a suspected or proven basal skull fracture should not be intubated nasally because of the possibility of intracranial placement of the endotracheal tube. However, recent data indicate that this complication is exceedingly rare and probably related to poor technique.

Patients with suspected or confirmed cervical spine injuries should be intubated with extreme caution, with every effort taken to avoid hyperextension of the neck. Intubation may be performed by either the oral or nasal route, preferably by an experienced intubator. If the orotracheal route is used, the intubator's assistant must provide "in-line traction" to prevent excessive extension of the neck. Intubation can also be achieved using a flexible bronchoscope or laryngoscope (by those experienced with the technique).

ENDOTRACHEAL TUBE SELECTION

The internal diameters of endotracheal tubes are usually measured in millimeters. Tubes are available in 0.5 mm increments from 2.5 mm. Selection of the correct size tube is of the utmost importance. The resistance to airflow varies with the fourth power of the radius of the tube. Selecting an inappropriately small tube increases the work of breathing. Furthermore, small tubes (less than 7.5 to 8.0 mm) will prevent bronchoscopic procedures from being performed through the endotracheal tube. Intubation with an inappropriately large tube may damage the larynx and vocal cords. In general, the larger the patient, the larger the endotracheal tube that should be used. Adult females should generally be intubated with a size 7.5 or 8.0 mm tube and adult males with an 8.0 or 8.5 mm tube.

ANESTHESIA FOR INTUBATION

When orotracheal intubation is attempted, it is crucial that the patient be adequately sedated to avoid fighting and airway trauma. If sedation alone does not result in adequate relaxation, an intravenous anesthetic induction agent alone or with a short-acting neuromuscular blocking agent can be used. It should be appreciated that both sedative and induction agents may precipitate severe hypotension in elderly patients and patients whose intravascular volume is depleted.

Sedation may be achieved using incremental doses of morphine sulphate (2 to 5 mg), fentanyl (100 µg), midazolam (2 to 5 mg), or lorazepam (1 mg). The combination of an opiate and a benzodiazepine is particularly effective in achieving adequate sedation. Thiopentone 100 to 300 mg or methohexital 50 to 150 mg can also be used. Succinylcholine (1 mg/kg), atracurium (0.5 mg/kg), or vecuronium (0.1 mg/kg) may be used for neuromuscular blockade. The latter has few hemodynamic effects and is relatively safe in patients with hyperkalemia and raised intracranial pressure. Pancuronium has a longer duration of onset and has a parasympatholytic effect, which may be undesirable in the already tachycardic patient. Lidocaine 1 mg/kg IV or fentanyl 100 to 200 µg given before intubation may blunt the sympathetic response to intubation.

The use of paralytic agents in patients who cannot be ventilated with a bag and mask may be fatal if intubation is unsuccessful. Therefore, paralytic agents should be used only by experienced intubators.

Hypotension is common after intubation and is best treated with volume replacement. Phenylephrine (Neo-Synephrine) is useful in patients who do not respond rapidly to fluids. One milliliter of phenylephrine (10 mg/ml) is diluted with 9 ml of NaCl and given in 0.5 to 1 ml boluses.

ENDOTRACHEAL INTUBATION

With the intubator standing behind the head of the bed, the initial step is to establish an airway by placing the finger of one hand under the mandible and lifting upward and backward (extending the patient's neck) or by using the index fingers of both hands to lift the mandible from the angle of the jaw. The ability to ventilate and oxygenate the patient with a bag and mask must then be established. Care should be taken not to generate excessive pressure when ventilating by bag and mask. Airway pressure exceeding 25 mm Hg is likely to overcome the resistance of the gastroesophageal sphincter and fill the patient's stomach with gas. This will increase the risk of regurgitation and gastric aspiration. When ventilation is effective, the chest rises with each squeeze of the bag. The patient should be preoxygenated in this way with 100% oxygen before intubation. Arterial oxygen saturation should be monitored continuously by pulse oximetry.

When an airway has been established and the patient adequately ventilated, preparation can be made for intubation. It is vitally important to assemble *all* the necessary equipment, drugs, and personnel at the bedside before attempting intubation. All the equipment must be inspected for completeness and tested for function. *As a general rule, a single operator should make no more than two attempts to intubate the trachea.*

If the second attempt is unsuccessful, ventilation of the patient's lungs with 100% oxygen should continue until more experienced help becomes available. Further attempts at intubation increase the risk of airway trauma and make subsequent attempts even more difficult.

OROTRACHEAL INTUBATION

- The intubator should wear gloves and a mask to protect himself or herself from potentially infectious agents, which may be transmitted during intubation.
- Perhaps the most important aspect of this technique is the correct positioning of the patient. The intubator should stand at the head of the bed. The patient must be in the supine position, with the height of the bed adjusted to achieve a comfortable position for the intubator. The patient's head should then be placed in the "sniffing" position, with the neck flexed and the head slightly extended. This is best achieved by placing a rolled bath towel under the occiput. It should always be assumed that the patient has a full stomach, and the Sellick maneuver (pressure applied to the cricoid cartilage) should be performed to prevent aspiration of regurgitated stomach contents into the trachea.
- The laryngoscope is grasped in the left hand while the patient's mouth is opened with the gloved right hand. The laryngoscope blade is inserted on the right side of the mouth and advanced to the base of the tongue, pushing the tongue to the left. If a straight blade is used, it should be extended below the epiglottis. If a curved blade is used, it is inserted in the vallecula.
- With the blade in place, the operator should lift the handle of the laryngoscope forward in a plane of 45 degrees to the horizontal to expose the vocal cords. It is essential to keep the left wrist stiff, and use the arm and shoulder to lift the laryngoscope. It is important to use a lifting action rather than to use the patient's teeth as a fulcrum to extend the head.

- The endotracheal tube is then held in the right hand and inserted into the right corner of the patient's mouth in a plane that intersects with the laryngoscope blade at the glottis. This angle avoids the problem of the endotracheal tube obscuring the view of the cords.
- The endotracheal tube is advanced through the vocal cords until the cuff just disappears from sight. If difficulty is encountered in advancing the tube through the cords, or when only the posterior portion of the cords is visible, it may be useful to use the introducing stylet. The soft metal stylet should be bent into the shape of a banana.
- *It should be emphasized that orotracheal intubation should not be performed if the cords cannot be seen. This is not a blind procedure.* If the vocal cords cannot be seen using a curved blade, a straight blade may facilitate visualization. In addition, firm cricoid pressure may bring the vocal cords into view.
- The cuff is then inflated with just enough air to prevent a leak during ventilation.
- The patient should be bagged with a CO_2 detector to confirm endotracheal placement of the endotracheal tube.
- The chest should be auscultated to ensure bilateral breath sounds.
- The tube should then be tied in position. The incisors should be at the 23 cm mark in men and the 21 cm mark in women.
- A portable chest radiograph should be obtained to confirm the position of the endotracheal tube and to exclude any complications that may have occurred during intubation.

NASOTRACHEAL INTUBATION

- The nares should be anesthetized with a topical anesthetic and a vasoconstrictor then applied.

- A 7.5 endotracheal tube is generally used. Warming the tube in hot water softens the tube and may allow for a less traumatic intubation.
- The endotracheal tube should be well lubricated. It is then inserted through the nares and gently advanced until breath sounds can be heard (with the intubator's ear near the end of the tube). The endotracheal tube is now positioned just above the cords. NOTE: The tube should be advanced gently. Using excessive force can cause severe upper airway trauma, including nasopharyngeal lacerations and rupture.
- As the patient takes a breath (and the vocal cords abduct) the tube is advanced through the cords and secured in position. If resistance is felt when advancing the tube, gentle flexion of the neck may correctly align the larynx.
- No more than two attempts at nasotracheal intubation should be made before the oral route is used.

THE DIFFICULT INTUBATION

The following features may suggest that intubation will be difficult:

- Short neck—chin to larynx distance (thyromental) less than three finger widths
- Obesity
- Protruding incisors
- Limited opening of mouth—interdental gap less than two finger widths
- Limited neck extension
- High, arched palate

However, many patients with none of these features also may be difficult to intubate. The most accepted method to assess the ease of intubation involves direct visualization of the oropharynx with the patient sitting and the tongue protruded. This type of assessment can rarely be made in an emergent situation.

THE FAILED INTUBATION

In those rare instances when an experienced intubator fails endotracheal intubation, fiberoptic bronchoscopic intubation may be successful. In the emergent situation, either a cricothyroidotomy or an emergent tracheostomy can be performed.

COMPLICATIONS ASSOCIATED WITH INTUBATION
Complications during intubation

- Arterial hypotension
- Upper airway trauma, including perforation or laceration of the pharynx, hypopharynx, or larynx
- Mainstem intubation
- Regurgitation with aspiration
- Arrhythmias and cardiorespiratory arrest
- Bleeding
- Esophageal intubation
- Cranial intubation

Delayed complications

- Sinusitis, otitis media, and pneumonia
- Tube blockage or kinking

Late complications

- Tracheomalacia
- Subglottic or tracheal stenosis
- Tracheoesophageal fistula
- Vocal cord paralysis

CHAPTER 2

Bronchoscopy

INDICATIONS

Flexible bronchoscopy has largely replaced rigid bronchoscopy as the procedure of choice for most endoscopic evaluations of the airway. Flexible bronchoscopy is easily performed, is associated with few complications, and allows greater visualization of the tracheobronchial tree than does rigid bronchoscopy. Despite these considerations, the indications for fiberoptic bronchoscopy in the ICU are limited and include the following:

- Atelectasis that has not improved despite aggressive physiotherapy.
- *Diffuse parenchymal disease in the HIV-positive patient*: bronchoscopy and bronchoalveolar lavage is the initial diagnostic procedure of choice in the HIV-positive patient with a diffuse alveolar infiltrate.
- *Diagnosis of ventilator-associated pneumonia*: bronchoscopy with protected specimen brush sampling or bronchoalveolar lavage together with quantitative culture is currently recommended as the procedure of choice for the diagnosis of ventilator-associated pneumonia.
- *Acute inhalational injury*: in patients exposed to smoke inhalation, fiberoptic laryngoscopy and bronchoscopy are indicated to identify the anatomic level and severity of injury.

- *The diagnosis of traumatic airway fracture*: after blunt trauma, patients who present with atelectasis, pneumomediastinum and/or pneumothorax may have sustained a fractured airway.
- *Foreign bodies*: forceps are available for use with the flexible bronchoscope, which may allow for the removal of foreign bodies.
- *Endotracheal intubation*: in difficult or failed intubations, the flexible bronchoscope may be used as an obturator for endotracheal intubation.

Rigid bronchoscopy is indicated for the removal of large foreign bodies, which may be difficult to remove with the flexible bronchoscope, and in the evaluation of patients with massive hemoptysis. Fiberoptic bronchoscopy has limited diagnostic value in the evaluation of the immunocompromised patient (except for HIV-positive patients) who present with respiratory failure and a bilateral pulmonary infiltrate. Fiberoptic biopsy and transbronchial biopsy have higher complication rates and lower diagnostic yields than open lung biopsy, which is the procedure of choice in this setting.

CONTRAINDICATIONS

- *Severe hypoxia*: on average, the PaO_2 will drop 20 mm Hg during bronchoscopy
- Poorly controlled asthmatics
- Hemodynamically unstable patients
- Unstable angina and postacute myocardial infarction
- Patients with high levels of PEEP

PERFORMANCE OF BRONCHOSCOPY

- *Sedation and anesthesia:* nonintubated patients should be lightly sedated with a short-acting benzodiazepine. It is important to ensure that the patient is calm and yet cooperative during the procedure. Local anesthesia is used to limit the irritation caused by the bronchoscope. Intubated, mechanically ventilated patients should be well sedated, since coughing during the procedure increases airway pressure, interferes with ventilation, and hampers the procedure. Because the endotracheal tube (or tracheostomy tube) bypasses the upper airways, local anesthesia is not required. Local anesthetic agents should not be used when performing protected specimen brush sampling.

- *Oxygenation*: it is essential that all patients be monitored with a pulse oximeter throughout the procedure and for several hours thereafter. Should the patient desaturate during the procedure, the bronchoscope should be removed immediately. Intubated, mechanically ventilated patients should be preoxygenated at 100%. The Fio_2 should remain at 100% during the procedure and for some hours thereafter because ventilation perfusion mismatching increases following bronchoscopy.

- Insertion of the bronchoscope

  In the nonintubated patient, the two standard approaches to the lower airways are transnasal and transoral. The transnasal approach has the advantage of virtually bypassing the gag reflex.

  An oral airway should be used when the bronchoscope is passed through the mouth, to prevent the patient from biting down on the bronchoscope.

  In the intubated patient, the bronchoscope is passed through the endotracheal tube. The endotracheal tube is fitted with an adapter, which allows for the simultaneous mechanical ventilation through one port and passage of the bronchoscope into the airway via the other. A size 8 (sometimes 7.5) or larger endotracheal tube is required both to ventilate the patient and to allow for the passage of the bronchoscope. In patients intubated with a smaller tube, a pediatric bronchoscope can be used, or the patient can be reintubated with a larger tube.

COMPLICATIONS

When performed by a trained specialist, flexible bronchoscopy is an extremely safe procedure. The complication rate increases significantly when transbronchial biopsy is performed. Complications include the following:

- Those associated with the use of sedation/anesthetic
- Hypoxemia
- Bleeding
- Vasovagal reactions
- Pneumothorax
- Pneumonia
- Bronchospasm
- Arrhythmias
- Acute myocardial infarction

CHAPTER 3

Normal values in pulmonary medicine

Table 3-1 Respiratory parameters

Abbre-viation	Parameter	Normal
RR	Respiratory rate	12-20
$Paco_2$	Arterial carbon dioxide tension	35-45 mm Hg
Pao_2	Arterial oxygen tension; $100 - \frac{1}{3}(\text{age} - 25)$	70-100 mm Hg
PAo_2	Alveolar gas tension	
	$PAo_2 = [Fio_2 \times (\text{Barometric pressure} - 47)] - Paco_2/0.8$	RA = 100 mm Hg
$AaDo_2$	Alveolar arterial o_2 difference $PAo_2 - Pao_2$	5-15 mm Hg
mVo_2	Mixed venous oxygen tension < 35 tissue hypoxia; < 30 severetissue hypoxia	35-40 mm Hg
P50	Pao_2 at which Hb is 50% saturated	22-30 mm Hg
TLC	Total lung capacity	4-6 L
VC	Vital capacity (IRV + ERV + TV) Female = $[27.63 - (0.112 \times \text{age})]$ $\times$ Height in cm Male = $[21.78 - (0.101 \times \text{age})]$ $\times$ Height in cm ± 50-80 ml/kg	> 75% predicted

Table 3-1 Respiratory parameters—cont'd

Abbre-viation	Parameter	Normal
FEV1	$\pm$40-60 ml/kg, decreases by 30ml/yr	> 80% predicted
FEV1/FVC		> 75% predicted
TV (V_T)	Tidal volume 6-7 ml/kg	
RV/TLC	Residual volume/total lung capacity ratio	< 0.3
Vd/V_T	Ratio of dead space to tidal volume	0.25-0.35
	Vd/V_T = (Pa_{CO_2} – PE_{CO_2})/Pa_{CO_2}	
PEFR	Peak expiratory flow rate, $\pm$10 L/kg/min	> 80% predicted
Cstat	Static compliance ($\Delta V/\Delta P$)	50-80 ml/cm H_2O
	Cstat = V_T/(plateau – PEEP); < 30 = "stiff lungs," < 20 ARDS	
Cdyn	Dynamic compliance = V_T/(peak pressure – PEEP)	
R_{AW}	Airway resistance (85% large airways)	
	R_{AW} = Peak pressure – plateau pressure	

CHAPTER 4

Respiratory failure and mechanical ventilation

There are two types of respiratory failure: type 1, Pao_2 < 55 mm Hg on room air, and type 2, Pao_2 > 45 mm Hg with Pao_2 < 55 mm Hg on room air.

The approach to patients with respiratory failure depends on the acuteness of the disorder, the blood gas determination, the nature of the disease causing the respiratory failure, and the patient's clinical condition. There are no strict rules about when a patient should be intubated; this is a clinical decision. In a patient with COPD on home O_2, it would be prudent to first attempt aggressive medical therapy before intubating the patient. The same would apply to an acute asthmatic in type 2 respiratory failure. On the other hand, a previously healthy patient with community-acquired pneumonia who remains hypoxic on 60% oxygen requires immediate intubation.

It should be emphasized that endotracheal intubation is not curative; it only buys time to allow correction of the underlying disorder. Endotracheal intubation and mechanical ventilation carry significant morbidity and mortality.

TYPES OF VENTILATORS

Ventilators have traditionally been classified according to the cycling method (cycling from inhalation to exhalation). However, modern ventilators have microprocessors, which allow them to function in many different modes with enormous versatility.

- *Volume cycled*: the ventilator delivers fresh gas until the preselected volume of gas is delivered. The rise in alveolar pressures is proportional to pulmonary compliance and the volume of gas delivered.
- *Pressure cycled*: inspiration continues until a predetermined peak airway pressure is reached. The tidal volume is variable (from breath to breath) and dependent on the following:
    Pulmonary compliance
    Respiratory rate
    Inspiratory time and flow rate
- *Time cycled*: inspiration continues for a preset interval, with exhalation beginning when this time interval has elapsed, regardless of airway pressure or volume delivered.

MODES OF VENTILATION (Fig. 4-1)

- *Controlled mechanical ventilation (CMV)*: the respiratory rate and tidal volume are preset. The patient cannot trigger the ventilator or move air through the ventilator circuit. The minute volume is therefore dependent on the preset respiratory rate and tidal volume. This mode of ventilation is only used in paralyzed patients.
- *Assist control (AC)*: in the AC mode, the ventilator senses an inspiratory effort by the patient and responds by delivering a preset tidal volume. The trigger threshold is the negative force that the patient must generate to trigger the ventilator. This trigger threshold can be adjusted, determining how hard the patient must work to trigger the ventilator. The trigger threshold is usually set at -2 cm H_2O. To prevent hypoventilation, a control mode back-up rate is set on the ventilator. If the time between two sponta-

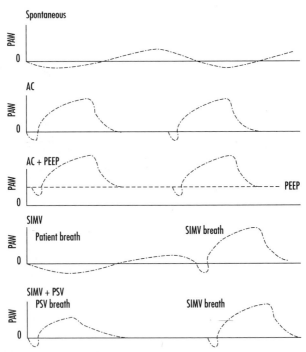

Fig. 4-1 Modes of mechanical ventilation.

neous inspiratory efforts is greater than the interval corresponding to the back-up rate, a breath of the same tidal volume is delivered.

- *Synchronized intermittent mandatory ventilation (SIMV)*: in the SIMV mode, the patient breathes spontaneously through the ventilator circuit at a tidal volume and rate that is determined according to the patient's needs. The patient, however, must open (trigger) a demand valve to breathe through the circuit, increasing the work of breathing. At regular intervals the ventilator delivers breaths based on a preset tidal volume and rate, which are synchronized with the patient's respiratory efforts. The degree of respiratory support is determined by the SIMV rate. SIMV theoretically has a number of advantages over AC ventilation.

Mean airway pressure is less, limiting the hemodynamic effects of positive pressure ventilation and reducing the risk of barotrauma

Hyperventilation and respiratory alkalosis are less likely

May maintain respiratory muscle strength
Patients may tolerate SIMV better than AC, requiring less sedation

SIMV may be used as a means of weaning the patient from mechanical ventilation

- *Pressure controlled ventilation (PCV)*: this is a form of AC ventilation. However, following patient or automatic triggering, the ventilator delivers a pressure-limited breath. The pressure above end-expiratory pressure is set, and the ventilator delivers a breath until this pressure is reached. As the pressure difference falls with progression of inspiration, the flow rate has a decelerating pattern. This inspiratory waveform has been shown to result in a more homogenous distribution of gas flow in patients with ARDS. The tidal volume varies (from breath to breath), being dependent on the set pressure, the compliance of the respiratory system, and the inspiratory time.
- *Pressure support ventilation (PSV)*: PSV was developed to reduce the work of spontaneous breathing in the SIMV mode. Each time the patient inhales, the ventilator delivers a pressure limited breath. The combination of PSV and SIMV permits the patient to breathe spontaneously while ensuring a minimal minute ventilation. PSV compensates for the inherent impedance of the ventilator circuit and endotracheal tube, enabling the patient to establish a more natural breathing pattern. A PSV of between 5 and 10 cm H_2O will overcome the resistance of the ventilator circuit and endotracheal tube.

PEEP

- PEEP provides *positive end-expiratory pressure* above atmospheric pressure. The mean airway pressure increases in proportion to the level of PEEP. In patients with pulmonary edema, PEEP shifts the pressure-volume inflation curve toward normal, increasing compliance, recruiting alveoli, and increasing FRC. It is thought that PEEP redistributes lung water. It should be recalled that PEEP decreases left ventricular afterload.
- *Physiologic PEEP*: some intensivists use "physiologic" or prophylactic PEEP (5 cm H_2O) to prevent atelectasis. Although recommended, there are no data to support or refute this practice.
- Indications
    Cardiogenic pulmonary edema
    Acute lung injury and ARDS
    Postoperative patients (decreased FRC)
- Contraindications
    Acute asthma
    Bullous lung disease and emphysema
    Raised intracranial pressure
    Unilateral lung disease (relative contraindication)
- *Best PEEP*: the level of PEEP that should be used is best PEEP. In patients with large intrapulmonary shunts, increasing the FiO_2 will not increase the PaO_2. However, excessive PEEP will overinflate compliant lungs and increase V/Q, mismatching as well as reducing cardiac output. A PEEP trial should be performed daily to determine the lowest level of PEEP that provides adequate arterial saturation and the maximal oxygen delivery.
- *PEEP valve*: when using more than 5 cm H_2O PEEP, a PEEP valve should be used when suctioning the patient. Disconnecting the endotracheal tube will result in a loss of PEEP, a rapid reduction in the FRC, and alveolar flooding.
- Detrimental effects of PEEP include the following:

Reduced venous return and cardiac output
Increased intracranial pressure
Reduction in hepatic and renal blood flow
Barotrauma
Increased intraabdominal pressure
Fluid retention
Increased inspiratory work load
Increased extravascular lung water
Alveolar overdistension and reduction in PaO_2
Ileus

- *Auto-PEEP*: as with spontaneous ventilation, exhalation during mechanical ventilation is a passive event and continues until the FRC is achieved. In patients with airflow limitation (asthma and COPD) and patients ventilated with reversed I:E ratios, a positive pressure breath may be initiated before exhalation is complete. This process leads to air-trapping and intrinsic or auto-PEEP. Auto-PEEP is common in mechanically ventilated patients. Auto-PEEP increases intrathoracic pressure, thereby exacerbating the effects of positive pressure ventilation. In patients with severe airflow limitation, severe auto-PEEP may develop. This may present with hemodynamic collapse similar to that of a tension pneumothorax. Auto-PEEP is treated by disconnecting the patient from the ventilator to "vent" the trapped air, and then changing the I:E ratio, allowing more time for exhalation. The presence of auto-PEEP cannot be detected unless the exhalation port venting to the atmosphere is occluded at end expiration (using a one-way valve). Some ventilators have an expiratory hold valve, enabling the auto-PEEP to be measured directly.

INSPIRATORY WAVEFORMS

Most ventilators offer at least three different types of inspiratory flow patterns in the SIMV and AC modes of ventilation. These include the following:

- A square wave, in which the inspiratory flow rises rapidly to a preset level and then stays at that level until the end of inspiration.
- A sinusoidal wave, in which the flow gradually increases and then decreases toward the end of inspiration.
- A descending ramp wave, in which the flow increases very rapidly and then decreases gradually until the end of inspiration. This pattern most closely mimics the normal inspiratory pattern.

In addition, the inspiratory wave can be modified by adjusting the inspiratory flow rate and inspiratory time and by providing an inspiratory pause (i.e., changing the I:E ratio).

INSPIRATORY TO EXPIRATORY RATIO

Some ventilators allow the operator to set the inspiratory to expiratory (I:E) ratio directly. Other ventilators allow adjustment of the I:E ratio by altering the flow rate, respiratory rate, and inspiratory time (including an inspiratory pause). For most adults a normal I:E ratio of 1:2 or 1:3 is used. In patients with chronic obstructive lung disease and asthma, longer I:E ratios are necessary to allow the lungs time to exhale to resting functional residual capacity and to avoid hyperinflation.

Patients who are hypoxemic secondary to ARDS require increased mean airway pressure to increase the FRC and allow more surface area for gas transfer to occur. This is achieved using both PEEP and inverse ratio ventilation. In addition, studies have demonstrated that prolonging inspiration can result in a more homogenous distribution of ventilation within abnormal lungs. By increasing the I:E ratio of 1:1 or more, the inspiratory pressure is maintained for a longer period. However, the peak inspiratory pressure does not increase.

INITIAL VENTILATOR SETTINGS (Fig. 4-2)

- AC or SIMV mode
- RR 12/min
- Tidal volume 8 ml/kg
- Peak flow 60 L/min
- Fio_2 90%
- I:E = 1:3
- ± PEEP 5 cm H_2O

MONITORING VENTILATED PATIENTS

- It is desirable that all patients receiving mechanical ventilation be monitored by pulse oximetry.
- Arterial blood gas analysis should be performed during the initial ventilator adjustments and then when clinically indicated. The arterial saturation, as measured by pulse oximetry and the venous pH and Pco_2, provides adequate information for managing most ventilated patients. Patients with CO_2 retention and patients with complex metabolic derangements generally require regular arterial blood gasses. It is not necessary to perform an arterial blood gas analysis after every ventilator change.
- All the ventilator parameters, including peak airway pressure, should be recorded on the patient's flow-chart hourly.
- The following formulas are useful in evaluating patients in respiratory failure:

  Age-predicted Pao_2 = Expected Pao_2 − 0.3 (age-25) [expected Pao_2 at sea level is 100 mg/Hg]

  As a general rule, expected $Pao_2 \approx Fio_2$ (%) × 5

  $AaDo_2$ = (FiO_2 × [BP* − 47]) − (Pao_2 + $Paco_2$/0.8)

---

*Barometric pressure.

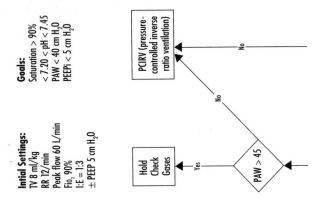

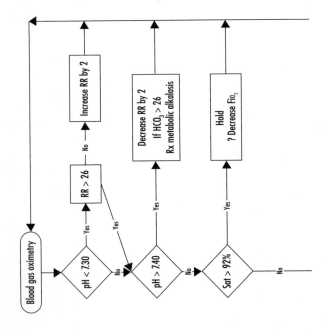

Intial Settings:
TV 8 ml/kg
RR 12/min
Peak flow 60 L/min
Fio_2 90%
I:E = 1:3
± PEEP 5 cm H_2O

Goals:
Saturation > 90%
$7.20 < pH < 7.45$
PAW < 40 cm H_2O
PEEPi < 5 cm H_2O

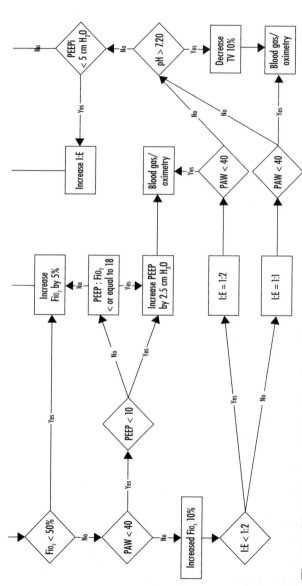

Fig. 4-2 Mechanical ventilation flow diagram.

The Pao_2/Fio_2 ratio is a better indicator of the degree of intrapulmonary shunting than the $AaDo_2$.

$$Vd/V_T = (Paco_2 - PEco_2)/Paco_2 \quad (N = 0.2\text{-}0.4)$$

SUDDEN INCREASE IN AIRWAY PRESSURE OR FALL IN ARTERIAL SATURATION

Causes

- Blocked endotracheal tube
- Herniated endotracheal tube cuff
- Tension pneumothorax
- Kinked endotracheal tube
- Tube migration (right mainstem bronchus)
- Mucous plug with lobal atelectasis
- Patient biting down on tube
- Patient ventilator synchrony

Management

- Administer 100% oxygen
- Check position of ET tube
- Suction through ET tube. If unable to pass catheter, then reintubate
- Auscultate chest for evidence of a pneumothorax; place chest drain immediately if chest is silent and trachea deviated
- Urgent chest x-ray
- If patient-ventilator asynchrony is likely, increasing the sedation may alleviate the problem. A patient should never be paralyzed until the cause has been determined

WHEN TO PERFORM A TRACHEOSTOMY IN THE VENTILATED PATIENT

There are no clear data to aid in the timing and indications of tracheostomy. The complication and infection rates appear to be similar when comparing long-term (up to 6 weeks) endotracheal intubation with tracheostomy. Indications (relative) for tracheostomy include the following:

- When prolonged endotracheal intubation is anticipated (i.e., > 14 days)
- Patients with neurologic diseases who are unable to protect their airway
- For bronchial toilet in patients who are unable to clear secretions
- Severe laryngeal edema or trauma from intubation

CHAPTER 5

Adult respiratory distress syndrome (ARDS)

DEFINITION, CAUSES, AND ASSESSMENT OF SEVERITY OF ALI

Acute lung injury (ALI) is a spectrum varying from mild ALI at one end to ARDS at the other. The diagnosis of ARDS should be reserved for patients with ALI who have severe disease (see criteria below). The outcome (and management) of ALI are largely dependent on both the severity of ALI and causative factors.

ALI is a condition involving the following:

1. An oxygenation defect with bilateral alveolar infiltrates
2. A patient who has suffered an acute catastrophic event
3. A patient with no underlying cardiopulmonary disease
4. A patient who has a pulmonary capillary wedge pressure ≤ 18 mm Hg or no clinical evidence of an elevated left atrial pressure

A patient is defined as having ALI when the $Po_2/Fio_2 \leq 300$ (regardless of the amount of PEEP). A patient is said to have ARDS when the $Po_2/Fio_2 \leq 200$ (regardless of the amount of PEEP).

Common causes of ALI and ARDS

- Sepsis and sepsis syndrome
- Pneumonia
- Trauma

- Pancreatitis
- Aspiration
- Drugs (heroin, tricyclic antidepressants)
- Fat embolism
- Smoke inhalation
- Chemical inhalation
- Drowning
- Posttransfusion
- Burns

MANAGEMENT OF THE ACUTE PHASE

Ventilation strategy

The ventilatory strategy (see Chapter 4 and Fig. 4-2) should be physiologically targeted and patient specific. The goals of ventilation are to maintain an arterial oxygen saturation above 90% and an arterial pH above 7.2. The lowest airway pressure that maintains adequate alveolar ventilation should be used (keep PAW below 40 cm H_2O and preferably below 35 cm H_2O). *Large tidal volumes overdistend compliant lungs, resulting in alveolar rupture and progressive lung injury.* In addition, if the patient is ventilated using a large tidal volume with low PEEP, derecruitment of lung units will occur with expiration. The following are recommended initial ventilator settings.

- *Low volume ventilation with permissive hypercapnia*: tidal volume of 5 to 7 ml/kg, adjusted to keep PAW less than 40 cm H_2O. This often results in an increase in $Paco_2$ and a fall in pH. The intracellular pH compensates more rapidly and completely than does the extracellular pH, and patients may tolerate an arterial pH as low as 7.2 (without a significant fall in myocardial contractility). Sodium bicarbonate should not be given because this increases CO_2 production, intracellular Pco_2, and intracellular acidosis. If intracellular acidosis is the determinant of reduced cardiac muscle performance, bicarbonate administration is more likely to be detrimental than beneficial.

- PEEP 8 to 10 cm H_2O, with titration, to keep the arterial saturation > 90%. "Best PEEP" should be used (see Chapter 4).
- I:E ratio should be 1:1.5. In patients with ALI, oxygenation is improved by increasing the mean airway pressure. This is achieved by both PEEP and inverse-ratio ventilation. By increasing the inspiratory time, the I:E ratio is increased; however, the peak airway pressure remains unchanged. The maximal benefit of inverse-ratio ventilation may take several hours to achieve. The respiratory rate must be adjusted to allow adequate time for expiration, thereby preventing excessive auto-PEEP. Auto-PEEP should be measured in all patients receiving inverse-ratio ventilation.
- Flow rate should be 50 to 60 L/min and adjusted to keep the PAW < 40 cm H_2O and to maintain I:E ratio.
- Fio_2 95%, with titration, to keep the arterial saturation > 90%.
- *Hemodynamics*: the lowest intravascular volume (or PCWP) that maintains an adequate cardiac index (and renal perfusion) should be achieved. Inotropic agents may be required to maintain the MAP > 70 mm Hg. If hemodynamics allow, the patient should be kept in a negative fluid balance. Once hemodynamic stability is achieved, the patient should be actively diuresed (until the BUN climbs to approximately 30 mg/dl). In patients with ALI, the higher the pulmonary capillary hydrostatic pressure, the greater the degree of capillary leak (and the greater the intrapulmonary shunt).
- *Optimizing oxygen transport*: it has been suggested that iatrogenically increasing oxygen delivery to predetermined levels may improve the outcome of patients with ARDS. There is little evidence to support this strategy. Oxygen transport should be titrated to tissue demands (see Chapter 53).
- *Pulmonary sepsis* (see Chapter 10): patients with ALI/ARDS have a high incidence of "secondary"

pulmonary infection. Pulmonary sepsis should therefore be aggressively diagnosed and treated.

- Supportive therapy

    GI prophylaxis (see Chapter 33)

    DVT prophylaxis (see Chapter 12)

    Maintain Hb > 7.5 g/dl

    Early enteral nutrition (if ileus, 20 ml/hr enteral nutrition and TPN)

    Correct coagulopathy, if patient is bleeding

    For intravascular catheters, change all intravascular lines every 8 to 10 days. Local erythema, increasing WBC, and/or unexplained temperature requires prompt removal of the catheter and replacement at a new site (see Chapter 42).

- *Tracheostomy*: if ventilation for longer than 14 days seems probable, perform tracheostomy as soon as feasible.
- Sedation (see Chapters 50 and 51)
- *Nitric Oxide*: inhaled nitric oxide acts as a selective pulmonary vasodilator when inspired at concentrations of 5 to 80 ppm. The rapid binding of nitric oxide to hemoglobin prevents systemic vasodilation. In patients with ARDS, inhaled nitric oxide will go preferentially to well-ventilated alveolar units, thereby diverting pulmonary blood flow away from the poorly ventilated alveoli to the better ventilated alveoli, with the net effect of decreasing intrapulmonary shunting. Controlled clinical trials are required to determine whether this therapeutic approach will improve patient outcome.
- *Extracorporeal respiratory support*: in randomized controlled clinical studies, extracorporeal respiratory support using either extracorporeal membrane oxygenation and carbon dioxide removal, or carbon dioxide removal alone, has been demonstrated to be of no benefit.
- *Corticosteroids*: prospective multicenter, placebo-controlled studies have demonstrated that high-dose

corticosteroids administered early in the course of ALI/ARDS are of no benefit. Patients treated with corticosteroids are at an increased risk of developing complications.

- *Other "experimental therapeutic modalities"*: the use of antioxidants, inhibitors of thromboxane and leukotrienes (NSAID, ketoconazole, etc.), prostaglandin E1, pentoxifylline, anticytokines, and exogenous surfactant, as well as many other therapeutic modalities, have not been proven to be of benefit in patients with ARDS and therefore cannot be recommended.
- There are no data to support the use of high-frequency jet ventilation in patients with ARDS. This ventilatory mode is fraught with problems and is potentially dangerous in patients with ARDS.

MANAGEMENT OF THE CHRONIC PHASE OF ARDS

After 10 to 14 days of aggressive supportive therapy, patients who require high levels of ventilatory support ($FiO_2 \geq 50\%$) are candidates for corticosteroid therapy. Corticosteroids should only be considered if lower respiratory tract sampling can be performed to diagnose and treat pulmonary sepsis. Some authors recommend an open lung biopsy before commencing corticosteroid therapy, in order to obtain histologic evidence of the fibroproliferative phase of ARDS and to exclude infection.

Before embarking on corticosteroid therapy, all possible sites of sepsis should be aggressively investigated and treated, i.e., intravascular and urinary catheters should be changed, and protected lower respiratory tract sampling and blood cultures should be performed. Once corticosteroids are commenced, vascular catheters should be changed, and surveillance cultures and protected lower respiratory tract sampling performed frequently (every third to fourth day).

CHAPTER 6

Weaning the patient from mechanical ventilation

WHEN TO WEAN

The concept of "weaning parameters" is a misnomer. The factors that need to be evaluated when considering weaning a patient from mechanical ventilation depend on the patient's underlying disease process and the reasons for intubation and mechanical ventilation in the first instance. For example, a healthy patient intubated because of a coma after a drug overdose can be extubated once that patient is awake and can protect the airway (measurements of respiratory muscle strength are of little value in this case). However, measurements of respiratory muscle strength are of vital importance in considering extubation in a patient with Guillain-Barré syndrome.

Factors to consider when weaning

- Improvement in the underlying disorder that required mechanical ventilation in the first instance.
- *Oxygenation*: Pao_2 above 60 mm Hg on 40% to 50% O_2. A Pao_2 of 55 to 60 mm Hg on 28% to 35% O_2 is acceptable in patients with chronic underlying lung disease. The Pao_2/Fio_2 should be > 200.
- *Alveolar ventilation*: a $Paco_2$ < 40 mm Hg in a patient with a minute ventilation less than 10 L. In patients with chronic underlying lung disease a $Paco_2$ > 40 mm Hg is acceptable as long as the minute ventilation is less than 10 L, the arterial pH is > 7.30, and

the patient is lucid and cooperative. A patient is unlikely to wean if the Vd/V_T is > 0.6 (see Table 3-1).

- *Respiratory muscle power*: it is important to assess respiratory muscle strength in patients with neuromuscular disorders and in patients who have undergone prolonged mechanical ventilation (because of muscle wasting).

  Negative inspiratory force (NIF) > 20 cm H_2O (maximal inspiratory pressure or MIP)

  Vital capacity > 10 ml/kg
  Tidal volume > 5 ml/kg

- *Respiratory muscle endurance*: it is important to assess this parameter in patients with neuromuscular diseases, in patients with chronic underlying lung disease, and in patients who have required mechanical ventilation for longer than 72 hours. An early sign of respiratory muscle fatigue is an increase in the respiratory rate and a fall in the tidal volume (when the patient is breathing unassisted by the ventilator).

  In general if the RR > 25 and/or the tidal volume < 4 ml/kg, it is unlikely that the patient will fare well with extubation. If the ratio of the RR to TV (in liters) is greater than 100, it is unlikely that the patient is weanable.

- Can the patient protect the airway? Does he or she have a gag reflex?

- *The cuff leak test*: this test is performed in patients suspected of having laryngeal edema. The cuff of the endotracheal tube is deflated; if there is no laryngeal edema, the patient should be able to breathe past the tube. A patient with a positive cuff leak test (i.e., no leak) has approximately a 30% chance of developing postextubation stridor; however, the risk is negligible in patients with a negative cuff leak test. The cuff leak test should be performed before extubation in the following circumstances:

  Traumatic intubation
  Prolonged intubation, i.e., longer than 5 to 7 days
  Patients with head and neck trauma

Head and neck surgery
Patients with previous failed extubation accompanied by stridor

METHODS OF WEANING

There is no right and wrong way to wean a patient. A review of the literature suggests that no one method is superior to another. Common "errors" in weaning include the following:

- Waiting too long before considering extubation
- Weaning a patient *too slowly*, once ready for extubation
- T-piece weaning with a small endotracheal tube (< size 8), especially in patients with cardiopulmonary disease. The greatest resistance in the ventilator circuit is the endotracheal tube (inversely related to radius^4). In addition, there is a loss of laryngeal PEEP (with reduction of FRC) when using a T-piece.
- Because of the increased work of breathing, patients *should not* be on a T-piece for longer than about 2 hours.
- The patient should be NPO for 6 hours before extubation, and the NG tube should be removed (to reduce the risk of aspiration). Don't forget to give IV glucose to prevent hypoglycemia.

Patients who have been ventilated for less than 5 days and patients with no underlying neuromuscular disorder can undergo a trial of spontaneous breathing through a T-piece circuit, with the Fio_2 set at the same level as that used during mechanical ventilation. The patient must be closely monitored during this trial. The trial should be terminated if the patient develops any of the following signs of respiratory distress:

- Respiratory rate > 35/min
- Arterial saturation < 90%
- Heart rate > 140 beats/min
- Systolic blood pressure > 180 mm Hg or < 90 mm Hg
- Agitation, diaphoresis, or anxiety

If the patient tolerates the T-piece trials, he can be extubated after 2 hours. If the patient fails this trial, he may be weaned by one of the following methods:

- Intermittent mandatory ventilation (+ PSV)
- Pressure support ventilation
- Intermittent trials of spontaneous breathing (T-piece trials)
- Once daily trials of spontaneous breathing (T-piece trials)

Synchronized intermittent mandatory ventilation (SIMV) with pressure support ventilation (PSV) is a convenient method of weaning patients with poor respiratory reserve from mechanical ventilation. The level of pressure support is set between 15 and 20 cm H_2O. The SIMV rate is then reduced incrementally to 0. The level of pressure support is then reduced incrementally, ensuring that the respiratory rate does not exceed 20 to 25/min. The level of pressure support should be reduced 5 to 8 cm H_2O (this level of pressure support overcomes the resistance of the endotracheal tube and ventilator circuit) before extubation.

T-bar weaning is performed by alternating increasingly long periods on the T-bar with full ventilation. During T-bar and SIMV (without PSV) weaning, the already fatigued muscle has to work against an increased work load (the ET tube and SIMV valves), causing further fatigue. Completely removing the work load (as with assist-controlled ventilation) is likely to lead to respiratory muscle atrophy (and hence weakness).

Pressure support efficiently assists each spontaneous breath by decreasing the respiratory work load imposed on the respiratory muscles. Monitoring the respiratory rate and the use of accessory muscles allows the physician to find a satisfactory work load for the patients, avoiding excessive loading on the one hand and total rest of the respiratory muscles on the other. This allows the respiratory muscles to recover and progressively increase their strength.

CHAPTER 7

Acute severe asthma

INDICATIONS FOR ADMISSION TO THE ICU

- Difficulty talking because of breathlessness
- Altered level of consciousness
- FEV1 and/or peak flow < 40% predicted
- Pulsus paradoxus > 18 mm Hg
- Pneumothorax or pneumomediastinum
- Pao_2 < 65 mm Hg on 40% O_2
- $Paco_2$ > 40 mm Hg
- Patient "tiring"

INITIAL TREATMENT

- Oxygen mask
- Beta$_2$-agonist by nebulization every 15 to 20 minutes initially, then 1 to 4 hourly
- *Corticosteroids*: methylprednisolone 60 mg IV q 6 hr
- Ipratropium bromide nebulization, q 2 to 4 hr, has synergistic bronchodilatory activity with beta$_2$-agonists
- *Theophylline (use controversial)*: if no ischemic heart disease and FEV1 and/or peak flow < 30% predicted and/or altered level of consciousness

  Theophylline has a narrow therapeutic index; therefore the serum level should be monitored in all critically ill patients

If patient is receiving maintenance theophylline, obtain a baseline theophylline level before starting theophylline

Loading dose 5 mg/kg given over 30 minutes (if not on maintenance theophylline)

Maintenance dose of 0.4 to 0.8 mg/kg/hr
0.4 mg/kg/hr in patients with COPD, heart failure, and liver dysfunction

0.06 mg/kg/hr in nonsmoking asthmatics
0.08 mg/kg/hr in asthmatics who smoke

Aim for theophylline level of 10 to 15 µg/ml

In refractory patients a level of 15 to 20 µg/ml may offer some therapeutic advantage. The dose response curve for theophylline is curvilinear. The level at which toxicity occurs is variable, however, and therefore all patients should be monitored for signs of toxicity.

- Do not use sedative drugs unless the patient is on a ventilator. If the patient has a large "psychosomatic" component to the asthma, and sedative drugs are deemed necessary, use small doses and observe closely in an ICU.

OTHER THERAPEUTIC OPTIONS

- IV or SQ beta$_2$-agonists
- SQ epinephrine 0.3 ml 1:1000 solution (drug of choice in anaphylactoid asthma). Epinephrine should be avoided in patients with a history of ischemic heart disease and/or hypertension.
- Ketamine infusion (sedative and bronchodilator)
- Heliox is a blend of helium and oxygen (80:20, 70:30, or 60:40) with a gas density approximately one third that of air. In normal subjects Heliox reduces R_{AW} by about 40% and increases maximum expiratory flows by about 50%. Heliox may be useful in "buying time" and avoiding intubation in acute attacks of asthma. In

mechanically ventilated patients with severe asthma, Heliox (60:40) has been demonstrated to reduce peak inspiratory pressure and $Paco_2$ by up to 50%.

The following should be noted:

1. General anesthesia (with halothane or enflurane) is probably of little value in the patient with a history of slowly worsening asthma (airway obstruction is predominantly the result of edema rather than bronchospasm).
2. SQ epinephrine may be useful in patients with severe asthma, especially if the onset is acute.

INDICATIONS FOR INTUBATION

Endotracheal intubation is not curative, is associated with significant morbidity, and can increase the degree of airway narrowing and inflammation. The timing of intubation is essentially one of clinical judgment. A high $Paco_2$ in itself is not an indication for intubation if the patient is alert and cooperative and the arterial pH > 7.2. The following are indications for intubation and mechanical ventilation:

- Altered consciousness
- Pao_2 < 50 mm Hg on a rebreathing mask
- Rising $Paco_2$ with a falling pH
- "Anaphylactic" asthma with rapidly deteriorating clinical course
- Patient fatigue

Blind nasal intubation is generally a safe method of intubation (beware of nasal polyps). Refer to Chapter 1.

MECHANICAL VENTILATION

- It is rarely a problem to oxygenate the patient with severe asthma; the problem is one of achieving adequate alveolar ventilation. The low dynamic compliance results in high airway pressures with the attendant risk of barotrauma. The resistance to expiration may result in significant auto-PEEP (iPEEP) with hemodynamic embarrassment. The goals of ventilatory therapy include the following:

Keep the peak airway pressure < 45 to 50 cm H_2O

Maintain arterial pH > 7.2

Limit iPEEP to < 5 to 10 cm H_2O

Do not use extrinsic PEEP (it has not been found to be useful)

Sedate the patient well; paralyze if necessary (avoid pancuronium, which causes histamine release and is vagolytic)

Adequate rehydration and maintain preload

- Initial ventilator settings

  Fio_2 60%

  Rate 12/min

  Peak flow 80 to 100 L/min

  Tidal volume 6 to 8 ml/kg

- The iPEEP and/or the exhaled tidal volumes must be measured in all patients to avoid significant air trapping. A low I:E ratio (long expiration) should always be used. Permissive hypoventilation should be used in patients with severe airway obstruction; however, the arterial pH should be kept above 7.20. Sodium bicarbonate boluses will make matters worse (increased intracellular CO_2 and acidosis) because of the fixed CO_2 elimination and should be avoided.

- If atelectasis occurs, it should be treated by aggressive chest physiotherapy. Bronchoscopy is potentially dangerous in intubated asthmatic patients.

- Monitor for barotrauma

CHAPTER 8

Acute respiratory failure in chronic obstructive pulmonary disease

Patients with chronic obstructive pulmonary disease (COPD) who acutely decompensate may benefit from admission to the ICU. Patients with end-stage disease with no acutely reversible or treatable condition should not be treated in an ICU.

COMMON PRECIPITATING EVENTS

- Upper respiratory tract infection
- Chest infection; acute bronchitis or pneumonia
- Pneumothorax
- Pleural effusion
- Pulmonary embolus
- Heart failure
- Arrhythmias
- Atelectasis/mucus plugging

Lower airway colonization by bacteria is common in patients with stable COPD. *Haemophilus influenzae, Streptococcus pneumoniae,* and *Moraxella catarrhalis* are the most common colonizing organisms. Approximately 30% of exacerbations of COPD are associated with viral infections, with influenza, parainfluenza, and respiratory syncytial virus being the most common etiologic agents. Recent studies using protected specimen brush sampling suggest that bacterial infection may be responsible for up to 50% of exacerbations of COPD. *H. influenzae, S. pneu-*

moniae, and *M. catarrhalis* were the most common pathogens. However, gram-negative rods (including *P. aeruginosa*) were isolated in a few patients. A Gram stain and culture should therefore be performed in all patients admitted to the ICU with an exacerbation of COPD (not to diagnose infection but to isolate the potential pathogens).

TREATMENT

- *Correct hypoxia*: this usually requires only small increases in Fio_2, i.e., 1 to 2 L by nasal cannula. *Avoid switching off the O_2 drive; keep Pao_2 at 55 to 60 mm Hg.* A high Pao_2 will decrease the respiratory drive in a patient with chronic CO_2 retention, with a potentially fatal outcome. Avoid endotracheal intubation and mechanical ventilation if possible; an elevated $Paco_2$ is acceptable as long as the patient is alert and cooperative, and the arterial pH is greater than 7.2. Recent studies suggest that in selected patients with an acute exacerbation of COPD, noninvasive ventilation can reduce the need for endotracheal intubation, the length of hospital stay, and the in-hospital mortality rate.
- Empiric antibiotics are often given to patients even if no obvious infectious precipitating cause is present. Cefuroxime, ampicillin/sulbactam, or azithromycin are suitable choices.
- Inhaled bronchodilators are usually given to all patients even if the patient does not have measurable reversible airway disease. $Beta_2$-agonists and ipratropium bromide should be used.
- A short course of intravenous corticosteroid therapy has been shown to be beneficial even in patients with no demonstrable airway obstruction.
- Theophylline may be useful in patients without ischemic heart disease (level of 10 to 15 µg/ml).
- SQ heparin

- Treat cardiac failure and electrolyte disturbances.
- *Chest physiotherapy*: directed at coughing and deep breathing, with chest percussion for atelectasis.
- Do not use sedative drugs unless the patient is on a ventilator.

For indications for and method of mechanical ventilation, refer to Chapter 7.

CHAPTER 9

Community-acquired pneumonia

- Causes of community-acquired pneumonia
  Streptococcus pneumoniae (50% to 70% of all cases)
  Mycoplasma pneumoniae
  Haemophilus influenzae
  Chlamydia pneumoniae (TWAR agent)
  Respiratory viruses
  Legionella sp.
  Staphylococcus aureus
  Moraxella catarrhalis
  Klebsiella pneumoniae
  Coxiella burnetii
  Neisseria meningitidis
  Escherichia coli
  Leptospira sp.

  In a third of cases no etiologic diagnosis can be made; many of these patients probably have pneumococcal pneumonia

- Causes of severe community-acquired pneumonia
  S. pneumoniae (probably 50% to 70% of all cases)
  Legionella sp. (0 to 30%)
  S. aureus (1% to 5%, especially during influenza epidemic)
  H. influenzae
  Klebsiella sp.
  Respiratory viruses
  Pseudomonas aeruginosa (very uncommon)

- Poor prognostic factors
    Age > 60 years
    $30 < WBC < 4 \times 10^9/L$
    BUN > 20 mg/dl
    Pao_2 < 60 mm Hg (room air)
    Multilobe involvement
    RR > 30/min
    Diastolic BP < 60 mm Hg
    Platelet < $80,000 \times 10^9/L$
- Noninfectious diseases masquerading as community-acquired pneumonia
    Bronchiolitis obliterans organizing pneumonia (BOOP)

    Eosinophilic pneumonia
    Hypersensitivity pneumonia
    Drug-induced pneumonitis: methotrexate, nitrofurantoin, gold, amiodarone

    Pulmonary vasculitis
    Pulmonary embolism or infarction
    Pulmonary malignancy
    Radiation pneumonitis
    Tuberculosis
- Microbiologic diagnosis
    Bronchoscopy and protected specimen brush sampling (or lavage) *before* commencing antibiotic therapy is probably the most sensitive and specific diagnostic method. *This is, however, extremely invasive and should rarely be performed.*

    Sputum Gram stain and culture has a sensitivity of about 20%, with a specificity of over 90%. This is an economical test and should be performed in all patients with pneumonia who have a productive cough. If the patient's cough is not productive, therapy should not be withheld until a specimen can be obtained.

    Blood cultures are positive in about 20% of patients with pneumococcal pneumonia and in less than

10% of patients with gram-negative pneumonia. Blood cultures should be drawn in all but the mildest cases of pneumonia.

TREATMENT (Fig. 9-1)

It should be noted that *S. pneumoniae* is still by far the most common pathogen isolated from patients with community-acquired pneumonia. Penicillin is the drug of choice for *S. pneumoniae* pneumonia, even if the organism is relatively penicillin resistant (low-grade resistance), because the serum concentrations far exceed the MICs. However, penicillin should not be used for organisms that demonstrate high-grade resistance. Currently in the United States, approximately 5% of *S. pneumoniae* cases are of low-grade resistance, and less than 1% are of high-level resistant. The resistance patterns, however, vary from one geographic region to another.

Persistent temperature

A common misconception is that the patient's temperature should settle within 24 hours of commencing antibiotic therapy. It has been demonstrated that it may take up to 72 hours for the temperature to normalize in a patient with pneumococcal pneumonia. However, in a patient with a widely swinging temperature, it would be prudent to exclude a complication within this time frame. The following are the major reasons for failure to respond to antimicrobial agents:

> Wrong antibiotic; wrong spectrum or drug resistance
> Wrong dosage
> Viral, fungal, or opportunistic pathogen
> Superadded complication
>> Complicated pleural effusion or empyema
>> Endocarditis
>> Purulent pericarditis
>> Septic arthritis
>> Meningitis

Complicated pleural effusion or empyema

When pleural fluid is detected in a patient with pneumonia, a diagnostic thoracocentesis should always be performed to rule out pleural space infection (except if the effusion is very small). Pleural fluid studies differentiate between a benign parapneumonic effusion and an early empyema (complicated pleural effusion). Chest tube drainage is necessary when the pleural fluid is grossly purulent or if pleural fluid studies show any of the following:

- pH < 7.2
- Glucose < 40 mg/dl
- White cell count > 10,000/ml

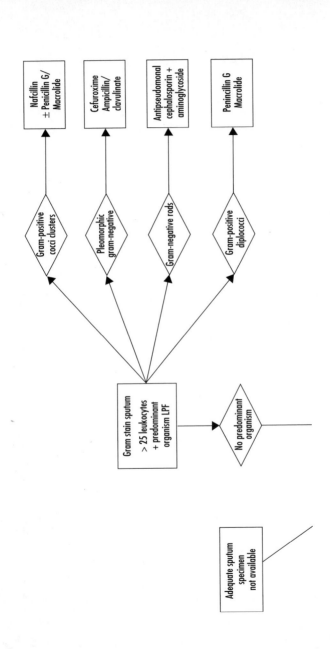

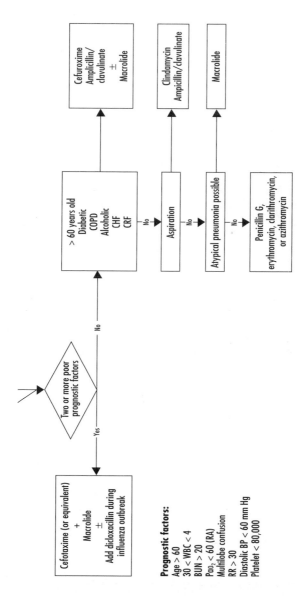

Prognostic factors:
Age > 60
30 < WBC < 4
BUN > 20
Pao₂ < 60 (RA)
Multilobe confusion
RR > 30
Diastolic BP < 60 mm Hg
Platelet < 80,000

Fig. 9-1 Empiric prescription for community-acquired pneumonia.

CHAPTER 10

Nosocomial pneumonia and ventilator-associated pneumonia

Pneumonia is a common complication in ICU patients, especially those undergoing mechanical ventilation. The optimal management of patients with suspected ventilator-associated pneumonia requires confirmation of the diagnosis and identification of the responsible pathogen or pathogens. Several recent studies have shown that the clinical criteria commonly used for diagnosing pneumonia are unreliable in acutely ill, ventilated patients, especially those with preexisting pulmonary infiltrates. Furthermore, colonization of the upper respiratory tract by potentially pathogenic bacteria limits the diagnostic value of Gram stain and culture of respiratory tract secretions. Bronchoscopic-directed sampling of lower respiratory tract secretions using a double sheathed protected specimen brush catheter and quantitative culture is currently considered the diagnostic method of choice in patients with suspected ventilator-associated pneumonia (Fig. 10-1).

The most common pathogens found in patients with ventilator-associated pneumonia include the following:

- *Pseudomonas aeruginosa*
- *Staphylococcus aureus*
- *Acinetobacter baumannii*
- *Klebsiella pneumoniae*
- *Escherichia coli*
- *Enterobacter cloacae*
- *Streptococcus agalactiae*
- *Streptococcus pneumoniae*
- *Haemophilus influenzae*

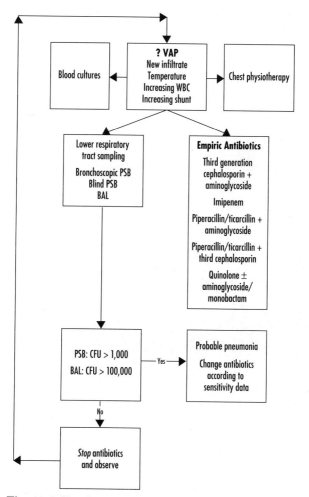

Fig. 10-1 Ventilator-associated pneumonia.

CHAPTER 11

Aspiration pneumonia

The approach to a patient with witnessed or suspected aspiration is dependent on the following:

- What is aspirated
- How much is aspirated
- The patient's local and systemic defense mechanisms
- The patient's level of consciousness
- The patient's oral hygiene and oropharyngeal flora

The interaction of the factors listed above will determine the nature of the aspiration syndrome.

- *Mendelson syndrome*: this syndrome is caused by the aspiration of liquid gastric contents. The volume and pH of the aspirated fluid are important pathogenetic factors. As little as 20 ml of gastric fluid with a pH < 2.5 is sufficient to cause this syndrome, which is characterized by a severe chemical pneumonitis and rapidly progressive ARDS.
- *Chemical pneumonitis syndrome*: this syndrome is caused by the aspiration of gastric contents whose pH and volume are insufficient to cause the Mendelson syndrome. These patients develop a noninfectious, self-limited pneumonitis and should be treated with supplemental oxygen. Steroids have not been proven to improve outcome. Antibiotics should not be given to patients with chemical pneumonitis (will select out resistant organisms). Antibiotics are indicated for superadded infections.

- *Pneumonia and lung abscess*: this usually occurs in patients with an altered level of consciousness and poor oral hygiene. Patients who are suspected to have aspirated under such circumstances should be treated with antibiotics, such as clindamycin, penicillin, or ampicillin/sulbactam.
- *Aspiration of undigested food*: this occurs in patients who vomit and are unable to protect their airway. It requires endotracheal intubation with suctioning. Flexible and/or rigid bronchoscopy may be required. These patients are at risk of developing pneumonia or abscess and should be treated with antibiotics.
- *Foreign body aspiration*: this is most common in children but may occur in adults with a depressed level of consciousness. These patients require rigid bronchoscopy and may require a thoracotomy.
- *Microaspiration of oropharyngeal contents in hospitalized patients*: this is the leading cause of nosocomial pneumonia.

_____

CHAPTER 12

Pulmonary embolus and deep venous thrombosis

DIAGNOSTIC ALGORITHM FOR PE

Refer to Fig. 12-1.

V/Q SCAN INTERPRETATION CATEGORIES
(Table 12-1)

- Normal and very low probability
  No perfusion defects
  ≤ Three small segmental defects with normal CXR
- Low probability
  > Three small segmental perfusion defects with normal CXR

  Large or moderate segmental perfusion defects involving > four segments in one lung, > three segments in one lung region with matching ventilation defects and normal CXR

  Nonsegmental perfusion defects
  One moderate segmental perfusion defect with normal CXR mismatch
- High probability
  ≥ Two large segmental perfusion defects without corresponding ventilation or CXR abnormality or with smaller ventilation or CXR abnormalities (mismatch)

  ≥ Two moderate segmental and one large segmental perfusion/ventilation mismatches

  ≥ Four moderate segmental perfusion/ventilation mismatches

Table 12-1 Probability of pulmonary embolus based on clinical suspicion and V/Q scan result

Lung scan interpretation	Prescan clinical suspicion	
	Any	High
High probability	0.87	0.96
Intermediate probability	0.3	0.66
Low probability	0.14	0.4
Normal	0	0.04

- Intermediate probability
  Includes all V/Q scans not listed in the previous categories

TREATMENT

- *Anticoagulation:* heparin should be started as soon as the clinical suspicion is raised, if no contraindications exist. The dose should be titrated to maintain a PTT of 2 to 2.5 times normal for 5 to 7 days (Table 12-2).

Table 12-2 Intravenous heparin monitoring and dosage adjustment

PTTs	Rate change (ml/hr)	Dosage change (U/24 hr)	Additional action	Next PTT
< 46	+5	+6000	Rebolus 5000 U	4-6 hr
46-54	+2	+2400	None	4-6 hr
55-85	0	0	None	Next morning
86-100	−2	−2400	Stop infusion 1 hr	4-6 hr after restart
>100	−5	−6000	Stop infusion 1 hr	4-6 hr after restart

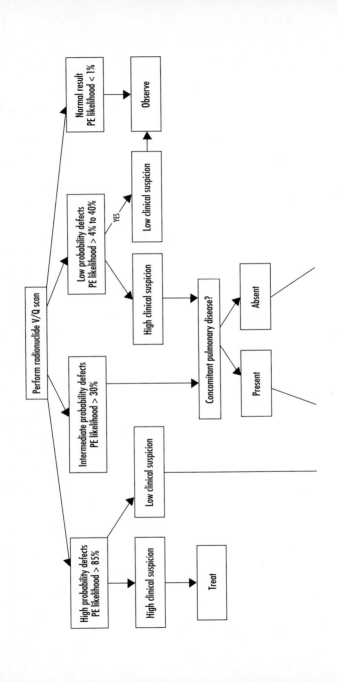

Perform radionuclide V/Q scan

- High probability defects
  PE likelihood > 85%
  - High clinical suspicion → Treat
  - Low clinical suspicion

- Intermediate probability defects
  PE likelihood > 30%

- Low probability defects
  PE likelihood > 4% to 40%
  - High clinical suspicion
  - Low clinical suspicion → Observe (YES)

- Normal result
  PE likelihood < 1% → Observe

Concomitant pulmonary disease?
- Present
- Absent

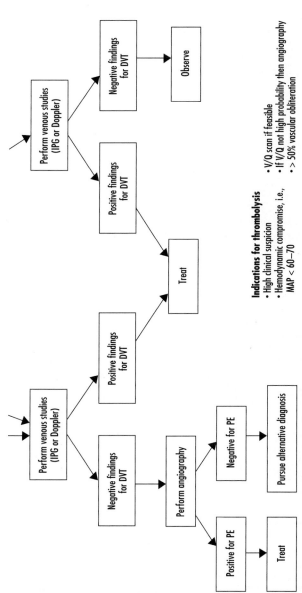

Indications for thrombolysis
- High clinical suspicion
- Hemodynamic compromise, i.e., MAP < 60–70
- V/Q scan if feasible
- If V/Q not high probability then angiography
- > 50% vascular obliteration

Fig. 12-1 Diagnostic algorithm for suspected pulmonary embolism (PE).

The single most common error in heparin therapy is underdosing (which leads to recurrent pulmonary emboli).

IV Heparin

Heparin 10,000 U bolus followed by 1250 U/hr (heparin 25,000 U in 500 ml DW infused at 25 ml/hr)

PTT in 6 hours (adjust according to Table 12-2) *SQ protocol:* heparin 10,000 U IV and 15,000 U SQ; then 15,000 SQ q 12 hr

- Once the PTT is stable (day 2 or 3) Coumadin 5 mg/day should be started. Heparin and Coumadin should overlap for 3 days. The dose of Coumadin should be adjusted to achieve an INR of 2.0 to 3.0 and given for at least 3 months.
- Thrombolytic therapy

Thrombolytic therapy should be considered in patients with acute massive pulmonary embolus who are hemodynamically unstable (hypotension, oliguria) and who have no contraindication to thrombolysis.

Thrombolytic therapy should also be considered in patients with greater than 50% obstruction of pulmonary perfusion on the lung scan.

Streptokinase is probably the drug of choice, with a loading dose of 250,000 U over 30 minutes followed by a continuous infusion of 100,000 U/hr for 24 hours, followed by heparin and Coumadin (as above).

- Indications for vena caval interruption

Patients in whom anticoagulation is contraindicated Failure of adequate anticoagulation to prevent recurrent pulmonary emboli

Patients in whom a further pulmonary embolus is likely to be fatal

Patients with heparin-associated thrombocytopenia

HEPARIN RESISTANCE

Heparin resistance has been arbitrarily defined as being present when a patient requires heparin in excess of 35,000 U/24 hr to achieve a targeted anticoagulant response. This may be due to reduced plasma concentrations of ATIII or increased concentrations of heparin-neutralizing proteins (histidine-rich glycoprotein, platelet factor IV, and vitronectin) or increased levels of procoagulants (particularly factor VIII). An increasing dose requirement that becomes evident during a course of therapy should raise suspicion of the development of the heparin-associated thrombocytopenia syndrome. Heparin resistance caused by low levels of ATIII may be successfully treated by the transfusion of 1 to 2 bags of fresh frozen plasma. Direct thrombin inhbitors (hirundin, hirulog) may prove to be useful in this setting.

High-dose intravenous nitroglycerin interferes with the anticoagulant properties of heparin. Nitroglycerin-induced heparin resistance may be a result of a qualitative ATIII abnormality.

HEPARIN-ASSOCIATED THROMBOCYTOPENIA (see Chapter 54)

Heparin should be stopped if the platelet count falls below 100,000.

DIAGNOSTIC ALGORITHM FOR SUSPECTED DVT (Fig. 12-2)

PROPHYLAXIS OF DEEP VEIN THROMBOSIS AND PULMONARY EMBOLUS (Table 12-3)

Risk Factors for DVT

- Previous PE/DVT
- Hip/pelvic surgery or trauma

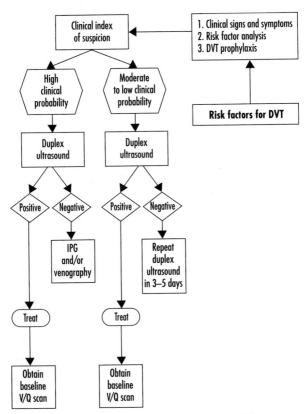

Fig. 12-2 Diagnostic algorithm for suspected deep venous thrombosis (DVT).

- Prostatic surgery
- Lower limb surgery or trauma
- Age > 60 years
- General surgery
- Obesity
- Cancer
- Estrogen-containing drugs

- Acute myocardial infarction
- Congestive cardiac failure
- Postpartum
- Prolonged bed rest

Table 12-3 Prophylactic therapy according to risk

Risk profile	Prophylactic therapy
Moderate risk	Low-dose heparin (LDH), 5000 U SQ q 12 hr or external pneumatic compression (EPC)
Moderate to high risk	
High-risk surgical patients	EPC *and* LDH or low molecular weight heparin (LMWH), 30 mg q 12 hr SQ
Neuromuscular paralysis in ICU and other high-risk ICU patients	EPC *and* LDH or LMWH
Neurosurgical procedures	EPC or LDH or EPC *and* LDH
Urologic surgery	EPC *and* LDH or LMWH
Multiple trauma	EPC or LMWH
Acute spinal cord injury	LMWH or adjusted dose heparin (ADH) to upper limit of normal range
High risk	
Total hip replacement	LMWH (started postperatively) *or* low intensity (INR 2.0-3.0) oral anticoagulation (started preoperatively *or* immediately after operation) or ADH (started preoperatively)
Total knee replacement	LMWH (started postoperatively)
Hip fracture surgery	LMWH (started preoperatively) or oral anticoagulation (INR 2.0-3.0) (started preoperatively)

PART TWO

THE CARDIOVASCULAR SYSTEM

CHAPTER 13

Cardiopulmonary resuscitation

GENERAL PRINCIPLES

- *Check abc: a*irways, *b*reathing, and *c*irculation.
- *Do not attempt* chest compressions on a conscious patient who is breathing and has a palpable pulse.
- In an unwitnessed cardiac arrest, try to determine how long the patient has been dead, e.g., temperature, lividity. *Do not attempt* to resuscitate a corpse.
- When running a code, it is essential that a single member of the team takes charge of the code and issues all the instructions.
- The femoral route is the simplest, quickest, and most direct method of obtaining central venous access. Do not try to cannulate the neck veins; you will obstruct the person ventilating the patient and the person performing chest compressions.
- Calcium chloride is no longer recommended during a code.
- The use of bicarbonate is controversial. Bicarbonate may be useful when the central venous pH < 7.2. Arterial pH values are misleading (Table 13-1).
- If spontaneous circulation cannot be established within 20 minutes, terminate the code.
- Data suggest that CPR is usually only successful in the setting of acute myocardial ischemia, primary arrhythmias, and other acutely reversible events (e.g., tension pneumothorax).

POOR PROGNOSTIC FEATURES

- Age > 60 years
- Unsuccessful out of hospital CPR
- Asystole
- Metastatic malignancy
- NYHA, class IV
- Renal failure
- Liver failure
- Pneumonia
- CPR > 15 minutes

TREATMENT OF VENTRICULAR FIBRILLATION

Refer to Fig. 13-1.

TREATMENT OF ASYSTOLE AND INDETERMINATE RHYTHM

Refer to Fig. 13-2.

DO-NOT-RESUSCITATE ORDERS

Refer to Chapter 46.

Table 13-1   Acid-base status and mVo_2 during CPR*

	Arterial gas	Mixed venous gas
pH	7.24	7.01
Pco_2 mm Hg	71	126
Po_2 mm Hg	107	29

*Mean values.

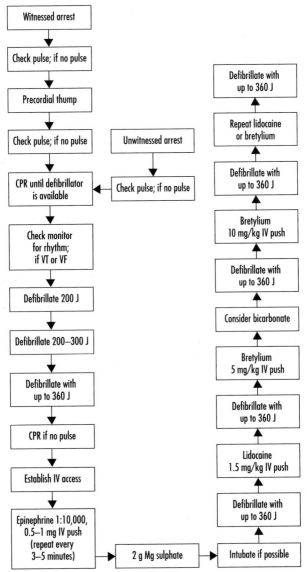

Fig. 13-1 Cardiac arrest—ventricular fibrillation (VF).

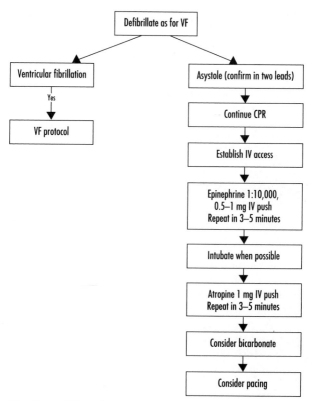

Fig. 13-2 CPR—rhythm unclear.

Hemodynamic monitoring and pulmonary artery catheterization

ARTERIAL PRESSURE MONITORING

The arterial blood pressure has traditionally been measured with a mercury sphygmomanometer and stethoscope. This time-honored method is reliable, reproducible, simple and economical, and is not associated with any major complications. The disadvantages of this method include operator variability, absence of Korotkoff sounds when the arterial pressure is low, and poor correlation with directly measured intraarterial pressure at the extremes of pressure. Automated manometer cuffs have been developed, which correlate well with the standard mercury sphygmomanometer.

Despite the proven reliability of the sphygmomanometer, over half of all patients admitted to an ICU have an arterial line inserted. With technologic improvements and a better understanding of the complications associated with intraarterial catheterization, the complication rates have been reduced. However, the complications associated with intraarterial catheterization are not minor and cannot be ignored. They include the following:

- Pain and swelling
- Arterial thrombosis
- Embolization
- Limb (digit) ischemia
- Catheter-related infection

- Hemorrhage
- Pseudoaneurysm
- Arteriovenous fistula
- Nerve damage
- *Excessive* diagnostic studies and blood loss

Indwelling arterial catheters result in excessive blood volume being taken for diagnostic tests and an excessive number of samples for blood gas analyses. Data suggest that the number of blood gas analyses performed on patients is related to the presence or absence of an arterial catheter rather than the clinical indications for such sampling.

Before the placement of an intraarterial radial catheter, an Allen test should be performed to confirm the patency of the ulnar artery.

Indications for intraarterial catheterization include the following:

- Patients in shock being treated with inotropic and/ or vasoactive agents, i.e., patients with a MAP < 60 mm Hg
- Hypertensive emergencies
- Patients who require 1 to 2 hourly blood sampling and/or patients with extremely poor venous access. With the widespread use of pulse oximetry, arterial blood gas analysis can be performed q 8 to 12 hours in all but the most unstable patients.

INDICATIONS FOR PULMONARY ARTERY CATHETERIZATION

Pulmonary artery catheterization (PAC) is a *diagnostic* rather than a therapeutic intervention, and as such, does not improve patient outcome. Recent data suggest that in a limited number of clinical settings, interventions that optimize the physiologic variables obtained from PAC *may* improve patient outcome. However, the complications associated with PAC and the incorrect determination or interpretation of the variables obtained may increase morbidity and mortality. In each patient the risk-benefit ratio of PAC needs to be carefully evaluated before the procedure is performed.

PAC may be useful in the following circumstances.

- Evaluation and optimization of intravascular volume status in:
    Refractory shock
    Acute renal failure
    Cardiogenic and noncardiogenic pulmonary edema
- Evaluation and optimization of the "hemodynamic and oxygenation profile" in the following:
    Acute myocardial infarction complicated by acute cardiac failure
    Septic shock
- Perioperative management of high-risk surgical patients
- Diagnostic catheterization
    To distinguish cardiogenic from noncardiogenic pulmonary edema

    To diagnose an acute ventricular septal defect

    Diagnosis and management of primary pulmonary hypertension

INSERTION OF A PAC

Central venous access is obtained as outlined in Chapter 58. It is easier to "float" a pulmonary artery catheter (PAC) from either the left subclavian or right internal jugular vein. Before inserting the PAC through the introducer, gently shake (jiggle) the tip and look at the waveform on the monitor; an undampened "sinusoidal" wave should appear. It is absolutely essential to ensure that an adequate waveform can be obtained before inserting the catheter. Also check the patency of the balloon.

The catheter is advanced through the introducer. Once the introducer is cleared (approximately 20 cm), the balloon should be inflated with 1.5 ml of air. The catheter is

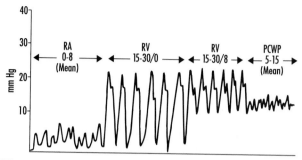

Fig. 14-1 Pressure tracing during insertion of a pulmonary artery catheter.

then advanced until the right ventricular tracing is obtained (approximately 30 cm from subclavian or internal jugular access). If the right ventricular tracing is not encountered, the balloon should be deflated and the catheter withdrawn into the central venous system. The catheter is then readvanced and the procedure repeated until a right ventricular tracing is obtained. Once the catheter is placed in the right ventricle, the catheter should be advanced into the pulmonary artery (an additional 10 to 15 cm) until a wedge tracing is obtained. The pressure waves obtained with insertion of a PAC are illustrated in Fig. 14-1.

COMPLICATIONS ASSOCIATED WITH PAC

The following minor and major life-threatening complications may follow PAC:

- Those associated with central venous access
- Arrhythmias during insertion
- Catheter-associated sepsis
- Balloon rupture
- Intracardiac knotting of the catheter
- Pulmonary infarction
- Pulmonary artery perforation

- Tricuspid and pulmonary valve damage and/or endo-carditis
- Cardiac perforation (with pacing electrode)
- Heparin-associated thrombocytopenia (from heparin bonding)
- Thrombotic and embolic complications

MEASUREMENT OF THE PULMONARY CAPILLARY WEDGE PRESSURE (PCWP)

In the critically ill patient the ongoing assessment of a patient's intravascular volume status is essential for optimal management. This seemingly simple evaluation may be clinically difficult, with PAC often performed for this indication. However, it is likely that as many as a third of all pressure readings are incorrectly determined or interpreted, resulting in incorrect therapeutic maneuvers. It is therefore important that all the following steps be diligently followed to minimize errors:

- The transducer must be zeroed to atmospheric pressure and fixed to a point that is level with the patient's fourth intercostal space in the midaxillary line (do not guess; use a builder's level, and mark the chest position for consistency).
- The dynamic compliance of the system should be checked. This is most easily done by using the rapid flush feature of the continuous irrigation device to provide a pressure signal that terminates abruptly. Observe the waveform on the screen. This procedure should produce a square waveform with an oscillating wave at the end of the waveform.

An overdamped system may be produced by the following:

Air bubbles
Kinking of the PAC or tubing
Too many stopcocks

Highly compliant tubing
Blood clots in the tubing
Tubing that is too long

An underdamped system may be produced by the following:

Tubing that is too short
Tubing that is too stiff

- The PCWP tracing should have the following characteristics:

    The PCWP cannot be greater than the pulmonary artery diastolic pressure.

    The phasic PCWP recording must be consistent with an atrial pressure waveform.

    The PCWP waveform should fluctuate with changes in intrapleural pressure.

A catheter wedged outside zone 3 of the lung will show marked respiratory variation, a smooth waveform, and misleadingly high pressures (PCWP > PA diastolic).

The PCWP should be determined visually using the freeze and cursor function of the oscilloscope or by obtaining a strip recording. The PCWP must be measured at end expiration and end diastole. It is critically important to identify end expiration on the PCWP tracing (*the waveform looks different after a spontaneous and a ventilator breath*). Isovolumetric ventricular contraction begins after the A wave at the onset of the C wave on the left atrial tracing. The AC wave junction (X′ descent) may be difficult to see on the PCWP tracing. Consequently, the top of the A wave or the mean PCWP can be used to estimate the left ventricular end-diastolic pressure (Fig. 14-2). When measuring the PCWP, it is important that the same reference point be used with each subsequent measurement to achieve consistency. Although convenient, the digital displays are inaccurate, uninterpretable, and totally misleading for determining the mean PCWP because of the

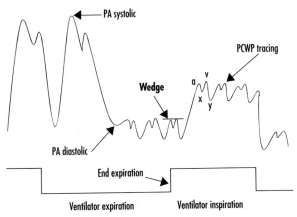

Fig. 14-2 Measurement of the PCWP.

unselective nature of the time-based electrical sampling and averaging. The digital readout is designed for arterial pressure monitoring only.

The PCWP is a measure of the pulmonary venous pressure (which determines the fluid flux across the pulmonary capillary membrane according to the Starling equation) and the left atrial filling pressure (and not left ventricular end-diastolic volume). The normal PCWP is 6 to 12 mm Hg and averages 2 to 5 mm Hg below the pulmonary artery diastolic pressure. In patients with a normal colloid osmotic pressure and intact pulmonary capillary membrane, interstitial pulmonary edema begins to develop with a wedge pressure above 18 to 20 mm Hg and florid intraalveolar edema with a PCWP above 25 mm Hg.

ERRORS IN THE INTERPRETATION OF THE PCWP

- PEEP (greater than 5 to 8 cm H_2O) increases intrapleural pressure (and intracardiac pressure) and therefore the pressure gradient between the left atrium (ventricle) and atmospheric pressure. This artifactually increases the PCWP. The "true" PCWP can only be determined if the intrapericardial pressure can be measured or estimated. Esophageal manometry may be useful in this instance. Formulas that subtract a percentage of the PEEP from the PCWP are of little value because the fraction of the PEEP that is transmitted to the heart is difficult to estimate.

- Pericardial tamponade and tension pneumothorax will increase the PCWP, while decreasing left ventricular end-diastolic volume.
- Changes in myocardial compliance will alter the PCWP and end-diastolic volume relationship. Myocardial ischemia decreases myocardial compliance, giving a higher PCWP for any given end-diastolic volume.
- The PCWP will not reflect left ventricular end-diastolic volume in patients with mitral stenosis and pulmonary venoocclusive disease.
- Patients with mitral incompetence will have a large CV wave, making interpretation of the PCWP difficult.

ANALYSIS OF MIXED VENOUS BLOOD SATURATION

Using the principles of pulse oximetry, PACs have been developed that can continuously measure the mixed venous oxygen saturation. Analysis of the mixed venous oxygen saturation can give an indication of cardiac output and tissue oxygenation. The normal mixed venous oxygen saturation is 70% to 75%. If cardiac output decreases, or if the oxygen demand increases, mixed venous oxygen saturation will fall. Continuous monitoring of the mixed venous oxygen saturation may therefore provide an early method of detecting inadequate tissue oxygenation.

DERIVED HEMODYNAMIC AND OXYGEN TRANSPORT VARIABLES

The simultaneous measurement of cardiac output, cardiac pressures, and arterial and mixed venous blood gas analysis will allow for the generation of an impressive number of derived physiologic variables. The formulas and normal values of these variables are listed in Table 14-1.

Pulmonary artery catheters equipped with a rapid response thermistor enable the computation of the right ventricular ejection fraction (RVEF). The end-diastolic and end-systolic volumes can be calculated as follows from the ejection fraction and stroke volume:

$$CO/HR \times 1000 = SV$$
$$SV/RVEF = RVEDV$$
$$RVEDV - SV = RVESV$$

The RVEDVI is an accurate measure of right ventricular preload. The "normal" range varies from 60-100 ml/M^2. A number of studies have demonstrated that the cardiac index is likely to increase with fluid loading when the RVEDVI is less than 90 ml/M^2 but unlikely to do so when the RVEDVI is greater than 140 ml/M^2. Furthermore, these studies have demonstrated that the cardiac index correlated better with the RVEDVI than with the PCWP. These data suggest that the RVEDVI more accurately predicts preload recruitable increases in cardiac index than does the PCWP.

It is important not to fall into the trap of treating numbers and forgetting to treat the patient (Table 14-2). Furthermore, as a consequence of the reproducibility error in the computation of the cardiac output, repeated measurements may differ because of the reproducibility error rather than representing real change. It has been demonstrated that two cardiac output measurements (mean of 3 determinations) should differ by more than *15% to 20%* to represent a real change.

Table 14-1 Measured and derived hemodynamic and oxygenation parameters

Parameter	Equation	Normal range
Mean arterial pressure (MAP)	From oscilloscope	70-105 mm Hg
Mean pulmonary artery pressure (MPAP)	From oscilloscope	10-20 mm Hg
PCWP	From oscilloscope	6-12 mm Hg
CVP	From oscilloscope	0-6 mm Hg
Cardiac output (CO)	From CO computer	4.0-8.0 L/min
Cardiac index (CI)	CO/BSA	2.6-4.0 L/min
Stroke volume (SV)	CO/HR	60-100 ml
Stroke index (SI)	SV/BSA	40-50 ml/M^2
R ventricular ejection fraction (RVEF)	From CO computer	40%-60%
R ventricular end-diastolic volume index	From CO computer	60-100 ml/M^2
L ventricular stroke work index (LVSWI)	$0.0136 \times SI \times (MAP - PCWP)$	50-62 gm.M/M^2
R ventricular stroke work index (RVSWI)	$0.0136 \times SI \times (MPAP - PCWP)$	5-10 gm.M/M^2
Systemic vascular index (SVR)	$(MAP - CVP) \times 80/CO$	800-1200 dynes.sec/cm^5
Systemic vascular resistance index (SVRI)	$SVR \times BSA$	2000-2400 dynes.sec/cm^5/M^2

Continued

Table 14-1 Measured and derived hemodynamic and oxygenation parameters—cont'd

Parameter	Equation	Normal range
Pulmonary vascular resistance (PVR)	$(MPAP - PCWP) \times 80/CO$	$100\text{-}250$ dynes.sec/cm^5
Pulmonary vascular resistance index (PVRI)	$PVR \times BSA$	$255\text{-}300$ dynes.sec/cm^5/M^2
Arterial O_2 content (CaO_2)	$(Hb \times 1.34 \times Sat) + (0.0031 \times PaO_2)$	$17\text{-}20$ ml/dl
Mixed venous O_2 content (CvO_2)	$(Hb \times 1.34 \times Sat) + (0.0031 \times PvO_2)$	$12\text{-}15$ ml/dl
Arteriovenous O_2 difference ($avDO_2$)	$CaO_2 - CvO_2$	$4\text{-}6$ ml/dl
Oxygen extraction ratio (O_2ER)	$avDO_2/CaO_2$	$20\%\text{-}30\%$
Venous admixture ratio (Qs/Qt)	$(CcapO_2 - CaO_2)/(CcapO_2 - CvO_2)$	$3\%\text{-}5\%$
Oxygen delivery (DO_2)	$(CO \times CaO_2)/10$	$950\text{-}1150$ ml/min
Oxygen delivery index (DO_2I)	DO_2/BSA	$500\text{-}600$ ml/min/M^2
Oxygen consumption (VO_2)	$(CO \times avDO_2)/10$	$200\text{-}250$ ml/min
Oxygen consumption index (VO_2I)	VO_2/BSA	$120\text{-}160$ ml/min/M^2

Table 14-2 Typical hemodynamic profiles obtained in various disorders

Diagnosis	CI	MAP	CVP	PCWP	SVRI	PVRI
Cardiogenic shock	↓	↓	↑	↑	↑	N-↑
Severe LV failure	↓	N-↓	N-↑	↑	↑	N
RV infarction	↓	↓	↑	N-↓	↑	N
Cardiac tamponade (PA diastolic = CVP = PCWP)	↓	↓	↑	↑	↑	N-↑
Severe mitral stenosis	↓	N-↓	↑	↑	↑	↑
Cor pulmonale	↓	N-↓	↑	N	↓	↑
Septic shock	↓-↑	↓	↓-↑	↓-↑	↓	↑
Hemorrhagic shock	↓	↓	↓	↓	↑	N-↑
End-stage liver disease	↑	↓	↓-↑	↓-↑	↓	N-↑
Massive PE	↓	↓	↑	N-↓	↑	↑

Resuscitation, hypotension, and fluid management

HYPOTENSION ALGORITHM

Refer to Fig. 15-1.

Marik's equation

Hypotension (or oliguria) + Clear chest = FLUID

After 1500 ml, stop and do the following:

- Reevaluate the patient (and diagnosis)
- Admit patient to the ICU
- Consider invasive hemodynamic monitoring

TYPE OF FLUID

The crystalloid vs colloid debate is a nondebate. Crystalloids essentially resuscitate the extravascular compartment, whereas colloids resuscitate the intravascular compartment. The type of resuscitation fluid will depend on the patient's clinical diagnosis and the volume status of each compartment. Most patients who have lost intravascular volume have lost both "colloid" (plasma) and "crystalloid" (intracellular and interstitial water). One should therefore replace both fluid types. Replacing only colloid may result in severe intracellular dehydration; replacing only crystalloid may result in excessive tissue edema.

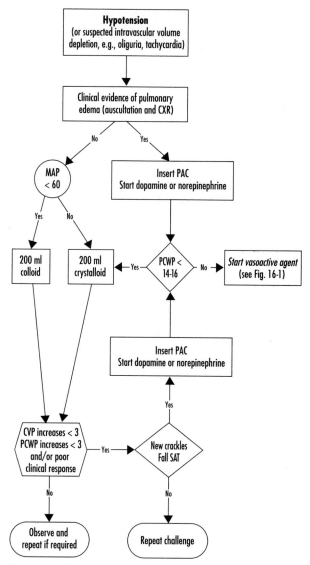

Fig. 15-1 Hypotension.

- *Hemorrhage*: fluid moves from the interstitial compartment to restore blood volume. Therefore both the intravascular and extravascular compartments are decreased. Hemorrhage models in animals have demonstrated a higher mortality when the animals are resuscitated with blood alone, compared with blood and crystalloids. Patients who have lost blood should therefore be initially rescuscitated with crystalloid and then with blood (and colloids).
- *Dehydration*: patients who are dehydrated (from diarrhea, vomiting, diabetic osmotic diuresis, etc.) have lost both intravascular and extravascular volume. Volume replacement with crystalloids will resuscitate both compartments.
- *Sepsis and the systemic inflammatory response syndrome*: (postoperative sepsis, trauma, or pancreatitis): as a consequence of "leaky capillaries" and "third-space loss," these patients have a decreased effective intravascular compartment and tissue edema. Since less than 20% of infused crystalloids remains intravascular in these patients, crystalloids should be used with extreme caution (see fluid balance in SIRS, p. 88).
- *Burns*: because of thermal injury, burn patients have a massive loss of interstitial fluid as well as a generalized capillary leak. Patients should be resuscitated with crystalloid during the first 24 hours.

As a general rule, patients should be resuscitated with a fluid similar to the type lost (Table 15-1), e.g., patients with diarrhea should receive 0.45 NaCl with supplemented

Table 15-1   Electrolyte content of body fluids

Type of loss	Na^+ mEq/L	K^+ mEq/L	HCO_3^- mEq/L
Gastric	40-80	5-15	—
Pancreatic	140-150	0-10	80-100
Bile	140-150	0-10	40-50
Ileostomy	120-140	5-20	30-60
Diarrhea	40-140	20-50	30-50

potassium and bicarbonate. Remember that no body fluid is more hypertonic than plasma.

CRYSTALLOIDS

Isotonic crystalloid solutions are safe and effective for the resuscitation of hypovolemic patients. Because isotonic fluids have the same osmolality as body fluids, there are no net osmotic forces tending to move water into or out of the intracellular compartment. The electrolytes and water partition themselves in a manner similar to the body's extravascular water content: 75% extravascular and 25% intravascular. Therefore three to four times the intravascular deficit is required. The partitioning occurs within 30 minutes of infusion, and within 2 hours, less than 20% of the infused liquid remains within the intravascular space (may be significantly less in patients with "leaky capillaries"). When compared with colloids, fluid exchanges with crystalloids are associated with only a small increase in cardiac output and oxygen delivery. Excessive administration of crystalloid is associated with pulmonary and generalized tissue edema.

- *0.9% NaCl*: this is the only crystalloid that can be mixed with blood. Patients may develop a hyperchloremic metabolic acidosis and/or hypernatremia.
- *Ringers lactate*: has a more physiologic electrolyte composition. The added lactate is converted to bicarbonate in the liver. This occurs readily, except in patients with profound liver dysfunction and "shocked liver."

COLLOIDS

These are solutions that rely on high molecular weight species for their osmotic effect. Because the barrier between the intravascular space is only partly permeable to the passage of these molecules, colloids tend to remain in the intravascular space for longer periods than do crystalloids.

Smaller quantities of colloids are therefore required to restore intravascular volume. Because of their oncotic pressure, colloids tend to draw fluid from the extravascular compartment into the intravascular space. The commercially available colloids have a mean molecular weight of about 70,000. Under conditions of normal capillary permeability, these molecules are ideally sized to remain in the intravascular space and contribute to the colloid osmotic pressure of serum.

- *Albumin*: this is available as a 5% solution. The serum half-life of exogenous albumin is less than 8 hours, though less than 10% leaves the vascular space within 2 hours of administration. After 2 days only 25% of the administered dose remains within the intravascular compartment. In patients with "leaky capillary syndrome," these molecules may leak from the intravascular space, lowering the colloid osmotic pressure of the plasma and drawing more fluid into an already compromised interstitium.
- *Hetastarch (Hespan)*: this is a synthetic hydroxyethyl starch, which is available as a 6% solution dissolved in normal saline. It is a polydispersed solution with molecular weights ranging from 10,000 to 2,000,000. The average molecular weight is approximately 69,000. About half the administered dose is excreted by the kidneys within 2 days and about 65% within 8 days. The large molecular weight moieties are taken up by the reticuloendothelial system and can be detected for as long as 42 days. Hetastarch may cause a thrombocytopenia and prolongation of the PTT because of an interaction of the large molecular weight moieties with platelets and factor VIII. The effects of hetastarch on intravascular volume expansion are similar to those of albumin. However, Hespan may be less likely to enter the extravascular space than albumin; the small MW moieties are excreted by the kidney, with the larger moieties remaining intravascular (Table 15-2).

Table 15-2 Constituents of common IV fluids

Fluid type	Na (mEq/L)	K (mEq/L)	Cl (mEq/L)	Lactate (mEq/L)	HCO$_3$ (mEq)	Osmolality (mosm/L)
5% glucose						278
NaCl 0.45%	77		77			154
NaCl 0.9%	154		154			308
Ringer's lactate	130	4	110	27		275
NaHCO$_3$ 4.2%	500				500	1000
NaHCO$_3$ 8.4%	1000				1000	2000
5% albumin	140		140			308
25% albumin	140		140			1500
6% hydroxyethyl starch	154		154			310

ENDPOINTS OF FLUID RESUSCITATION

One needs to tread a very cautious path because underresuscitation may result in acute tubular necrosis, and overzealous fluid replacement may result in generalized tissue and pulmonary edema (see also Chapter 14).

- The best clinical endpoint is urine output. The kidney is an excellent barometer of intravascular volume. Aim for an initial urine output of 0.5 to 1 ml/kg/hr.
- The CVP is an extremely poor endpoint for fluid resuscitation. Studies have demonstrated *no correlation* between the CVP and either the blood volume or the right ventricular end-diastolic volume (Fig. 15-2). In fact the CVP may fall with fluid resuscitation (because of decreased autonomic tone). Therapy guided by the CVP is likely to result in fluid overload and/or pulmonary edema.
- *Pulmonary artery catheterization*: many of the limitations to the use of the CVP apply to the PCWP (a poor indicator of intravascular volume and left ventricular end-diastolic volume). The "Ref catheter" (right ventricular ejection fraction pulmonary

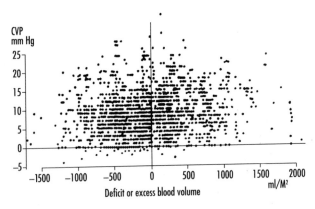

Fig. 15-2 Plot of blood volume and CVP (from Shippey CR et al: *Crit Care Med* 12:107, 1984).

artery catheter) allows for the computation of the right ventricular end-diastolic volume. A number of studies have shown this to be a useful determinant of intravascular volume and recruitable cardiac index.

- In patients with ongoing bleeding, one should aim for a MAP > 60 and a urine output of about 0.5 ml/kg/hr until the cause of bleeding has been treated (the higher the MAP, the greater the blood loss until the cause has been treated). This will avoid overresuscitation.

Recent data suggest that patients who are hypotensive and have suffered traumatic injuries *should not be fluid resuscitated* until the cause of bleeding has been surgically corrected, i.e., should not be fluid resuscitated at the site of injury or in the ER (patients should only be cannulated). Fluid resuscitation would therefore only begin in the OR. It is suggested that fluid resuscitation dislodges clots, dilutes coagulation factors, and increases the rate of bleeding (as a result of a higher MAP). This therapeutic approach is supported by both experimental studies and clinical trials.

CLINICAL SIGNS OF INADEQUATE TISSUE PERFUSION

- Hypothermia
- Hypotension
- Oliguria
- Altered sensorium
- Peripheral cyanosis
- Skin mottling
- Cold extremities
- Cold knees (Marik sign); temperature gradient between the thigh and the knee

THE TREATMENT OF HYPOALBUMINEMIA

Hypoalbuminemia is a common finding in critically ill patients. It has been well documented that hypoalbuminemic patients have a higher morbidity and mortality than patients with a normal serum albumin. Consequently, hypoalbuminemic patients are commonly treated with exogenous albumin in the hope of improving their outcome. A review of the prospective, randomized studies, which have been reported to date, do not support this practice. The administration of albumin for the purpose of raising reduced serum levels has been described by Rosenoer and Rothschild in *Albumin structure, function, and uses* (Pergamon Press, 1977, p. 4) as the "ultimate metabolic misunderstanding."

One of the major motivations for the use of albumin in the critically ill patient has been to prevent pulmonary and tissue edema by enhancing the plasma COP. However, in the critically ill patient there is a very poor relationship between the serum albumin and COP. Furthermore, endothelial injury with "leaky" capillaries (reduced σ in the Starling equation) is common in critically ill patients, reducing the importance of the COP in influencing fluid flux. Albumin supplementation has only a transitory effect on the serum albumin concentration because of the redistribution of albumin from the intravascular to the extravascular space. Contrary to common belief, only about 40% of the total body albumin is intravascular.

The only circumstances in which the treatment of hypoalbuminemia with exogenous albumin has been proven to be of benefit are when it is combined with a loop diuretic in cirrhotic patients with refractory ascites, large volume paracentesis, and in nephrotic patients with anasarca.

FLUIDS IN THE CAPILLARY LEAK SYNDROMES: ALI (acute lung injury), ARDS, AND SIRS (systemic inflammatory response syndrome)

Vascular endothelial injury with "leaky" capillaries is common in critically ill patients. Many factors, including sepsis, major surgery, trauma, burns, and pancreatitis, result in white cell and immunomediated endothelial damage. This process results in "third-space" fluid loss. The degree of fluid loss depends on the severity of the endothelial damage as well as the number of vascular beds involved. The hydrostatic pressure in the vascular bed becomes a major determinant of the fluid flux across the endothelial membrane. That is, for any hydrostatic pressure, the movement of fluid across the capillary bed will be greater in leaky capillaries than it will in normal ones.

A positive fluid balance is characteristic of this phase of tissue injury (Fig. 15-3). Fluid loading is essential to maintain intravascular volume and an adequate cardiac output. A vasoconstrictor (norepinephrine) may be useful to limit the amount of fluid required to maintain adequate tissue perfusion. An attempt to diurese patients during this phase of the disease may result in serious hemodynamic compromise. The type of fluid that should be used to maintain

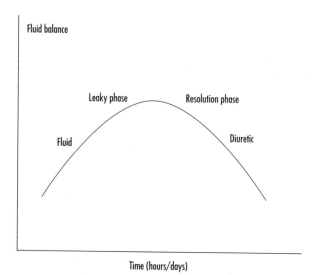

Fig. 15-3 Fluid balance in leaky capillary syndrome.

intravascular volume in this situation is unclear. Theoretically, a colloid with large molecular weight molecules should limit the degree of fluid leak. This speculation, however, remains unproven.

Once the capillary endothelial injury begins to resolve, the "third-space" tissue edema will begin to be absorbed. Diuretics are useful during this phase to facilitate this process.

It is essential to realize that fluids are required during the "leaky" phase and diuretics during the resolution phase. Diuretics during the "leaky" phase may lead to vascular collapse. Theoretically, agents that limit the degree of endothelial damage may shorten the duration of the "leaky" phase.

CHAPTER 16

Adrenergic agonists and antagonists

CHOICE OF INOTROPIC AGENTS

Refer to Fig. 16-1.

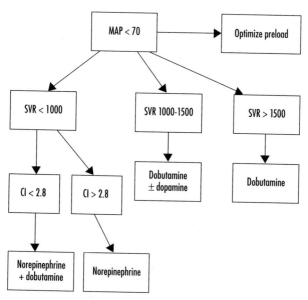

Fig. 16-1 Inotropic agents and hypotension.

- Dobutamine is the drug of choice to increase myocardial contractility.
- Norepinephrine is the drug of choice to increase systemic vascular resistance.
- "Low-dose" dopamine increases renal blood flow and may have a role in oliguric states (see Chapter 27).
- Epinephrine is the drug of choice for anaphylactic shock, "anaphylactic" asthma, and during resuscitation of a patient with cardiac arrest.
- Dobutamine and norepinephrine may be a useful combination in patients with depressed contractility (low LVSWI), low cardiac index, together with a low systemic vascular resistance, i.e., patients with underlying heart disease who develop sepsis or patients with myocardial depression caused by sepsis.
- There are very few indications for phenylephrine in the critically ill patient. Very few disease processes respond favorably to a fall in cardiac index. Furthermore, the relatively long half-life of this drug makes dose titration difficult.

Refer to Tables 16-1 to 16-3.

Table 16-1 Inotropic agents: receptor occupation and hemodynamic effects

	Epinephrine	Norepinephrine	Dopamine	Dobutamine	Phenylephrine
Alpha-1	+++	++++	++ (Third)	+	+++
Alpha-2	++	++++	++	+	0
Beta-1	++++	+++	+++ (Second)	++++	0
Beta-2	++	0	+	++	0
Dopamine (DA1 and DA2)	0	0	+++ (First)	0	0
Cardiac index	+++	+	+++	++	−
HR	+++	+	+++	++	+/−
SVR	+/−	+++	+/−	−	+++
LCWI	+++	++	+++	++	++
O$_2$ consumption	++	0/+	++	+	0
Blood glucose	+++	0/+	+	+	0

Table 16-2 Beta-blockers

Drug	ISA*	Beta-1 selective	Lipid solubility	$T_{\frac{1}{2}}$(hr)	Total daily initial	Usual dosages (mg)‡
Acebutolol	+	+	Low	3-4	200-400	400-800
Atenolol	–	+	Low	6-9	25-50 (5 IV bolus)†	50-100
Labetalol	?	– (alpha)	Low	3-4	100-400 (5-20 IV bolus)†	5000-1000 (q 6-12 hr)
Metoprolol	–	+	Intermediate	3-4	25-50 (5 IV bolus)†	50-200 (q 12 hr-qd)
Nadolol	–	–	Low	14-24	40-80	40-160
Pindolol	++	–	Intermediate	3-4	5-15	10-15 (q 12 hr-qd)
Propranolol	–	–	High	3-4	10-80 (1 mg IV)†	80-240 (q 6 hr-qd)
Sotalol	–	–	Low	8-10	80	160 (q 12 hr-qd)
Timolol	–	–	Low	4-5	5-10	10-20 (q 12 hr-qd)

*ISA, Intrinsic sympathomimetic activity.
† Patients may be given a single IV bolus of the beta-blocker in the dosage indicated, together with an oral dose. Sometimes it may be necessary to repeat the loading dose. Refer to Table 16-3 for labetalol and esmolol dosage infusion rate.
‡ Dosage refers to the total daily dosage and *not* the divided dosages (the daily dosage should be halved for an q12 hr dosage interval).

Table 16-3 Cardioactive drugs: dosage and preparation

Drug	Loading dose	Maintenance dose	Preparation
Adenosine	3-12 mg		
Amiodarone	5-10 mg/kg	5 µg/kg/min	300 mg/250 ml D_5W
Amrinone	0.75 mg/kg	5-10 µg/kg/min	400 mg/250ml 0.9 NaCl
Bretylium	5-10 mg/kg	0.5-4 mg/min	2000 mg/250 ml D_5W
Clonidine	0.1-0.2 mg PO	0.1-0.3 mg q 12 hr	Oral
Diltiazem	0.15-0.25 mg/kg	2-3 µg/kg/min	125 mg/250 ml D_5W
Dobutamine	Titrate to effect	2-20 µg/kg/min (max 60)	500 mg/250 ml D_5W
Dopamine	Titrate to effect	2-20 µg/kg/min (max 60)	400 mg/250 ml D_5W
Epinephrine	Titrate to effect	0.05-2 µg/kg/min	2 mg/250 ml D_5W
Esmolol	500 µg/kg	50-200 µg/kg/min	2.5 g/250 ml D_5W
Isoproterenol		1-10 µg/min	2 mg/250 ml D_5W
Labetalol	5-20 mg	2-3 mg/min	300 mg/250 ml D_5W
Lidocaine	1mg/kg	1-4 mg/min	2 g/500 ml D_5W
Magnesium sulphate	1-2 g	1-2.5 g/hr	25 g/250 ml D_5W

Continued

Table 16-3 Cardioactive drugs: dosage and preparation—cont'd

Drug	Loading dose	Maintenance dose	Preparation
Milrinone	50 mg/kg	0.25-1 mg/kg/min	30 mg/250 ml D_5W
Nicardipine	5 mg/hr increase by 2.5	to max 15 mg/hr	
Nimodopine	10 μg/kg	0.5 μg/kg/min	
Nitroglycerin		5-50 (100) μg/min	100 mg/250 ml D_5W
Nitroprusside		0.5-2 (10) μg/kg/min	100 mg/250 ml D_5W
Norepinephrine		0.03-0.6 μg/kg/min	8 mg/250 ml D_5W
Phenylephrine	100-200 μg	2-10 μg/kg/min	30 mg/250 ml D_5W
Procainamide	50-100 mg every 5 min up to total dose of 17 mg/kg	2-6 mg/min	1000 mg/250 ml D_5W
Propranolol	1-3 mg	3-8 mg/hr	20 mg/250 ml D_5W
Trimethaphan		3-6 mg/min	500 mg/250 ml D_5W
Verapamil	1 mg/min up to 20 mg	1-5 μg/kg/min	50 mg/250 ml D_5W

CHAPTER 17

Hypertensive emergencies and management of hypertension in the ICU

HYPERTENSIVE EMERGENCIES

Indications for the emergent reduction of a markedly elevated blood pressure (diastolic > 120 mm Hg)

- Hypertensive encephalopathy and/or papilledema
- Dissecting aortic aneurysm
- Acute pulmonary edema with respiratory failure
- Acute myocardial infarction or unstable angina
- Eclampsia

*These are the **only** indications for the immediate and rapid reduction of a markedly elevated blood pressure.* In patients who have suffered a major cerebrovascular event, the blood pressure *should not* be immediately lowered (may cause further cerebral ischemia). In all other patients the blood pressure can be lowered slowly using oral agents.

MANAGEMENT OF HYPERTENSIVE EMERGENCIES

The blood pressure in patients with hypertensive emergencies should be treated in a controlled fashion in an ICU. *This disorder should not be treated in the emergency room.* The use of sublingual nifedipine or IM hydralazine must be *strongly condemned*. The patient should be admitted to an ICU as an emergency case, and the blood pressure should be reduced in a controlled fashion using an infusion of nitroprusside, labetalol, or nicardipine (a dihydropyridine calcium channel blocker). Intraarterial blood pressure monitoring is essential.

- Patients with cerebral edema are probably best treated with labetalol or nicardipine, because nitroprusside has been shown to increase intracranial pressure (ICP).
- Patients with an acute myocardial infarction or angina are probably best treated with labetalol (or esmolol) ± nitroprusside. Esmolol is a cardioselective beta-blocker with a short half-life (10 minutes), allowing easy titration.
- Patients with acute pulmonary edema are probably best treated with nitroprusside or nicardipine.
- Patients with a dissecting aneurysm should receive an infusion of nitroprusside *and* a beta-blocker (labetalol, esmolol, propranolol) to reduce the arterial wall shear force.
- Patients with eclampsia are probably best treated with $MgSO_4$ and an IV infusion of hydralazine (*not* IM). Nicardipine, although untested, may be useful in this condition. Low doses of labetalol or nitroprusside may be used with caution.*
- Patients receiving nitroprusside should be monitored for evidence of cyanide toxicity (see p. 99).

Contrary to popular belief, nitroglycerin is not an effective vasodilator. Nitroglycerin is a potent venodilator and only affects arterial tone at high doses. Nitroglycerin reduces blood pressure by reducing preload and cardiac output.

---

*It should be noted that $MgSO_4$ is used for the treatment and prophylaxis of seizures and is not an antihypertensive agent.

NITROPRUSSIDE-RELATED CYANIDE POISONING

Nitroprusside contains 44% cyanide by weight. Cyanide is released nonenzymatically from nitroprusside, the amount generated being dependent on the dose of nitroprusside administered. Cyanide is metabolized in the liver to thiocyanate. Thiosulfate is required for this reaction. Thiocyanate is 100 times less toxic than cyanide. The thiocyanate generated is excreted largely through the kidneys. Cyanide removal therefore requires adequate liver function, renal function, and bioavailability of thiosulfate.

Cyanide toxicity has been documented to result in unexplained cardiac arrest, coma, encephalopathy, convulsions, and irreversible focal neurologic abnormalities. The current methods of monitoring for cyanide toxicity are insensitive. Metabolic acidosis is usually a preterminal event. A rise in serum thiocyanate levels is a late event and not directly related to cyanide toxicity. RBC cyanide concentrations (although not widely available) may be a more reliable method of monitoring for cyanide toxicity. A RBC cyanide concentration above 40 nmol/ml results in detectable metabolic changes. Levels above 200 nmol/ml are associated with severe clinical symptoms, and levels greater than 400 nmol/ml are considered lethal. Data suggest that nitroprusside infusion rates in excess of 4 µg/kg/min, for as little as 2 to 3 hours, may lead to cyanide levels that are in the toxic range. The recommended dosages of nitroprusside of up to 10 µg/kg/min result in cyanide formation at a far greater rate than human beings can detoxify.

It is therefore recommended that nitroprusside be avoided in patients with significant hepatic or renal dysfunction, that the duration of treatment be as short as possible, and that the infusion rate should not exceed 2 µg/kg/min. An infusion of thiosulfate should be used in patients receiving higher dosages (4 to 10 µg/kg/min) of nitroprusside. It has also been demonstrated that hydroxocobalamin (vitamin B_{12a}) is safe and effective in preventing and treating cyanide toxicity associated with the use of nitroprusside. This may be given as a continuous infusion at a rate of 25 mg/hr. Hydroxocobalamin is unstable and should be stored dry and protected from light. Cyanocobalamin (vitamin B_{12}), however, is ineffective as an antidote and is not capable of preventing cyanide toxicity.

ENDPOINTS OF THERAPY

The immediate goal of IV therapy is to reduce the diastolic blood pressure by 10% to 15% or to about 110 mm Hg. In patients with a dissecting aneurysm this goal should be achieved within 5 to 10 minutes. In other patients this endpoint should be achieved within 30 to 60 minutes. In patients with long-standing hypertension the cerebral blood flow autoregulatory range is shifted to the right (Fig. 17-1). The rapid and uncontrolled reduction of blood pressure will result in cerebral and renal ischemia or infarction. Once the endpoints of therapy have been reached, the patient can be started on oral maintenance therapy.

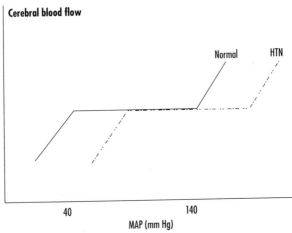

Fig. 17-1 Cerebral blood flow autoregulation.

MANAGEMENT OF THE HYPERTENSIVE PATIENT IN THE ICU

It is important to determine the cause of the patient's hypertension. Does the patient have a history of hypertension? ICU patients may be hypertensive because of agitation, pain and anxiety, volume depletion, or drug and alcohol withdrawal.

There are a large number of agents that can be used for the control of hypertension in the ICU. These drugs can be used orally, intravenously, or transdermally. Diuretics are generally not recommended (in the ICU) for the control of blood pressure.

- Calcium channel blockers are useful antihypertensive agents. Sublingual nifedipine should be avoided because of its unpredictable pharmacodynamic effect. Nicardipine is the only dihydroperidine calcium channel blocker currently available in an intravenous form.
- Beta-blockers are effective drugs for the control of hypertension in the ICU patient. They may be used orally or intravenously.
- ACE inhibitors are useful agents for the treatment of hypertension in patients with LV dysfunction and in diabetic patients. Chronic renal failure is *not* a contraindication to their use. This class of drugs, however, should be avoided in patients with acute renal dysfunction or azotemia. Enalapril is available in both an oral and intravenous formulation. ACE inhibitors are absolutely contraindicated in patients with bilateral renal artery stenosis and patients with moderate to severe aortic stenosis.
- Clonidine (PO, transdermal) is a useful third-line agent. This drug is often effective in treating hypertension associated with cocaine abuse and alcohol withdrawal.

CHAPTER 18

Cardiac failure
in the ICU

Patients with end-stage cardiac failure should not be admitted to an ICU unless they have suffered an acute reversible event or are candidates for cardiac transplantation.

- Unless contraindicated, patients should be treated with a combination of digoxin, an ACE inhibitor, and a diuretic. Clinical trials have confirmed that monotherapy with diuretics, digoxin, or ACE inhibitors is not satisfactory for NYHA class II patients in sinus rhythm who have an ejection fraction of less than 35% and who have overt heart failure. Renal function should be closely monitored, because a subgroup of patients will have a fixed cardiac output, and renal function will decline precipitously after instituting an ACE inhibitor.
- In those patients in whom ACE inhibitors are contraindicated or cause adverse effects, the addition of isosorbide dinitrate and hydralazine to the therapeutic regimen of digoxin and diuretics has been demonstrated to have a favorable effect on left ventricular function and mortality.
- In patients with angina, the combination of digoxin, diuretic, and nitrate is preferable because ACE inhibitor therapy has been shown to cause an increase in angina in these patients.
- ACE inhibitors are *contraindicated* in patients with moderate to severe aortic stenosis, bilateral renal

artery stenosis, hypertrophic obstructive cardio-myopathy, and pericardial tamponade.

- Symptoms and signs of pulmonary edema should be treated with repeated doses (IV) of a loop diuretic. Patients with cardiac failure require a high filling pressure (Starling principle), and excessive diuresis may compromise cardiac output.
- Metolazone (Zaroxolyn 5 to 20 mg PO daily) acts synergistically with loop diuretics and may be useful in patients who have not responded to a loop diuretic alone. Monitor the serum potassium because this combination of drugs can cause severe hypokalemia.
- Small doses of morphine sulphate (1 to 2 mg) are useful in alleviating anxiety (also decreases preload). Large doses may suppress the respiratory drive, resulting in worsening hypoxemia.
- Patients *may* benefit from a short course of dobutamine.
- Patients with pulmonary edema may benefit from positive pressure ventilation with PEEP or nasal CPAP/ BiPAP. Positive pressure ventilation is good for the left side of the heart. It reduces the work of breathing and LV afterload.
- The preload should be optimized.
- The use of beta-blockers in the treatment of cardiac failure is controversial. Beta-blockers have been shown to be of benefit in "stable" patients with idio-pathic dilated cardiomyopathies. They should not be used in patients who have acutely decompensated unless the patients have severe diastolic dysfunction. The progressive increase in the dose of the beta-blocking agent appears to be an important factor allowing hemodynamic and functional benefit in patients with heart failure. Studies have shown that improvement in ejection fraction takes several months to develop. In contrast the nonprogressive adminis-tration of antihypertensive doses of beta-blockade often leads to hemodynamic as well as functional status deterioration. This suggests that beta-blockers *should not* be used in patients with acute decompen-

sated cardiac failure but rather in "stable" patients already receiving maximal medical therapy.

- ACE inhibitors have been demonstrated to be useful in patients with moderate to severe aortic incompetence and in patients with mitral incompetence.
- Patients with obstructive cardiomyopathy may benefit from "apical pacing."
- DVT prophylaxis
- The use of low-dose amiodarone in patients with congestive cardiac failure is controversial. It appears that amiodarone may reduce the mortality in patients with idiopathic dilated cardiomyopathies but not in patients with congestive cardiac failure caused by coronary artery disease. Confirmation of this observation is required before this therapy can be widely recommended.

DIASTOLIC DYSFUNCTION IN HEART FAILURE

Diastolic dysfunction is defined as "decreased diastolic distensibility (compliance) of the left ventricle." Myocardial fibrosis, hypertrophy, ischemia, and aging predispose a patient to diastolic dysfunction. Although there is some degree of diastolic dysfunction in most patients who present clinically with heart failure, as many as 40% of patients with congestive heart failure have normal systolic function and thus have primary diastolic failure. In these patients the left ventricle is nondilated and contracts normally, but ventricular diastolic function is greatly impaired. In these patients relatively small increases in end-diastolic volume, resulting from even mild sodium and water overload, may lead to exaggerated increases in end-diastolic pressures, and pulmonary edema may develop despite normal or even reduced end-diastolic volumes.

Chronic systemic hypertension is the commonest condition predisposing a patient to diastolic dysfunction. Myocardial ischemia and elevated afterload (aortic stenosis) are other common causes. Patients with "small hearts" or unexplained symptoms of cardiac failure should undergo echocardiography to confirm the diagnosis. Occult coronary artery disease should also be excluded.

Beta-blockers or calcium channel blockers appear to be the most efficacious agents (alone or with diuretics) in the management of patients with cardiac failure resulting *primarily* from diastolic dysfunction. Direct-acting vasodilators are poorly tolerated in these patients. The role of ACE inhibitors is unclear at this time.

Unstable and stable angina

UNSTABLE ANGINA

Patients with unstable angina may benefit from admission to an ICU with aggressive medical treatment. The therapeutic plan needs to be individualized according to the patient's cardiac and clinical status. Treatment will include the following:

- Aspirin 1 stat, then daily
- IV nitroglycerin titrated to the patient's pain and blood pressure (40 to 400 µg/min)
- Full anticoagulation with IV heparin
- Beta-blockade, titrated to pulse and according to LV function. Typical dosages of beta-blockers in myocardial ischemia include the following:
    Propranolol 40 to 80 mg q 6 hr; 1 mg IV q 5 min × 3
    Metoprolol 50 to 100 mg q 12 hr; 5 mg IV × 2
    Timolol 10 to 20 mg q 12 hr
    Atenolol 50 to 100 q day, 5 mg IV × 2
    Esmolol 500 µg/kg IV then 50 to 200 µg/kg/min infusion
- Strict bed rest
- An anxiolytic
- Calcium channel blockers, such as diltiazem, may have a role in patients with ongoing chest pain
- Morphine is particularly beneficial in treating pain, allaying anxiety and reducing preload

STABLE ANGINA

Canadian cardiovascular classification of angina

- *Class 1*: pain is precipitated only by severe and usually prolonged exertion.
- *Class 2*: pain on moderate effort (e.g., precipitated by walking uphill or by walking briskly for more than three blocks on the level, in the cold, against wind, or provoked by emotional stress). There is slight limitation of ordinary activity.
- *Class 3*: marked limitation of ordinary activity; pain occurs on mild exertion, usually restricting daily chores. Patient is unable to walk two blocks on the level at a comfortable temperature and at a normal pace.
- *Class 4*: chest discomfort on almost any physical activity.

Medical therapy

- Aspirin
- Beta-blockers
- +/− calcium channel blockers in patients with normal LV function
- Diet, an exercise protocol, and cholesterol lowering agents

Angioplasty

Indications for angioplasty

- Patients with stable class 2 or class 3 angina
- Ejection fraction greater than 40%
- Acceptable angiographic lesions

And

- Inadequate control of angina with medical therapy
- Proximal single vessel disease with 70% to 90% stenosis
- Double vessel disease, without high-grade LAD stenosis

Indications for coronary revascularization surgery (coronary artery bypass grafting)

- Triple vessel disease
- Left main disease
- Double vessel disease with proximal LAD disease
- Male sex and age < 65 years (there are no data to indicate that bypass surgery is better than medical therapy in female patients and patients over the age of 65 years)

CHAPTER 20

Acute myocardial infarction (AMI)

RISK STRATIFICATION

Refer to Tables 20-1 to 20-3.

Table 20-1 Killip classification of acute myocardial infarction

Class	Definition
I	No rales and no S3
II	Rales < 50% lung fields or S3
III	Rales > 50% lung fields
IV	Cardiogenic shock

Table 20-2 Forrester classification of acute myocardial infarction

Class	PCWP (mm Hg)	CI (L/min)	Mortality (%)
I	< 18	> 2.2	3
II	> 18	> 2.2	9
III	< 18	< 2.2	23
IV	> 18	< 2.2	51

Table 20-3 In-hospital mortality risk stratification

Parameter	Approximate mortality (%)
Average	13
Age: 75-85	24
65-74	15
50-64	9
< 50	< 7
Cardiogenic shock	80
Large anterior AMI with the following:	
Severe CHF	> 30
Previous AMI and EF < 30%	> 25
Q wave AMI with HR > 100 and SBP < 110	> 20
New LBBB	> 20
Anterior Q wave AMI uncomplicated	12
Inferior Q wave AMI	3
Non-Q wave	3
Q wave and age < 55 uncomplicated	7
Non-Q wave age < 55	1

THROMBOLYTIC THERAPY AND PHARMACOLOGIC INTERVENTIONS IN ACUTE MYOCARDIAL INFARCTION

Refer to Tables 20-4 to 20-7.

Heparin protocol for fibrin-specific activators

The TIMI 9 and GUSTO IIa studies have shown that unless the PTT is closely monitored and the upper limit of the PTT is reduced, there is an excessive incidence of intracranial bleeding. Hence, when using heparin and fibrin-specific activators, the PTT must be closely monitored and kept in the range of 55 to 80 seconds.

Table 20-4 Summary of the mega-AMI studies

Trial	Control	SK	t-PA	Beta-blocker	Aspirin	H+SK	H+t-PA	ACE	NTG
MIAMI	4.9			4.3					
GISSI I	13	10.7							
GISSI II		8.5	8.9						
		22.8	22.9			22.2	23.3		
GISSI III	7.2							6.6	7.0
ISIS I	4.57			3.89					
ISIS II	12.2	9.2			9.4				
ISIS III		10.6	10.7			10.5	10		
ASET	9.8		7.9						
ISAM	7.1	6.3							

Shaded area, combined endpoints of severe CHF and death; *H*, heparin; *SK*, streptokinase; *NTG*, nitroglycerin.

Continued

Table 20-4 Summary of the mega-AMI studies—cont'd

	Short-term mortality (%) (2-6 weeks)								
Trial	Control	SK	t-PA	Beta-blocker	Aspirin	H+SK	H+t-PA	ACE	NTG
GUSTO						7.2	6.3		
LATE:									
6-12 hr	11.9						8.7		
12-24 hr	9.2						8.7		
EMERAS:									
7-12 hr	12.8	11.3							
12-24 hr	10.8	11.0							

Shaded area, combined endpoints of severe CHF and death; *H*, heparin; *SK*, streptokinase; *NTG*, nitroglycerin.

Table 20-5 Dosages of thrombolytic agents

Agent	Dosage
Conventional t-PA	100 mg or 1 mg/kg for those < 65 kg over 3 hr with 10% of the dose given as an initial bolus
Front-loaded t-PA	100 mg over 1.5 hr with 15 mg initial bolus
Streptokinase	1,500,000 IU over 1 hr
APSAC	30 mg over 2-5 min

Table 20-6 Dosages of beta-blockers in AMI

Agent	IV	IV 1-7 days	Oral After first week
Atenolol	5 mg over minutes, repeated 10 min later	10 min after last IV dose 50 mg	50 mg
Metoprolol	5 mg over 5 min, repeated 5 min later and again 5 min later	8 hr after IV dose 25-50 mg q 12 hr	50-100 mg q 12 hr
Propranolol	*Not FDA approved*	20 mg q 8 hr	80 mg LA up to 160 mg LA
Timolol	*Not FDA approved*	5 mg q 12 hr	10 mg q 12 hr

Table 20-7 Heparin and fibrin-specific activators in AMI*

	Patency of infarct related vessel (%)	Mortality (%) (30 day)
Heparin	79.5	5.5
No heparin	56.7	9.2

*Summary from a number of studies.

- Bolus of 5000 U
- Infusion at 1000 U/hr (heparin 25,000 U in 500 ml DW infused at 20 ml/hr)
- PTT in 6 hours (adjust according to Table 20-8)
- Continue for 3 to 5 days

It should be noted that high-dose intravenous nitroglycerin interferes with the anticoagulant properties of heparin.

Contraindications to thrombolysis

- Absolute contraindications
    Active peptic ulcer with recent bleeding
    Suspected aortic aneurysm
    Recent head injury or cerebral neoplasm
    CVA within the last 2 months
    Trauma or major surgery within the last 6 weeks
    Recent prolonged or traumatic CPR
    Diabetic retinopathy or other ophthalmic hemorrhagic lesions
    Acute pancreatitis
    Pregnancy
    Severe hypertension, B/P > 200/100 mm Hg
- Relative contraindications
    Active peptic ulcer without bleeding and being treated
    Minor trauma or surgery beyond 2 weeks
    Severe hypertension with B/P > 180/100 mm Hg
    Significant liver dysfunction or esophageal varices
    Underlying malignancy
    Elderly patients who are lethargic, confused, or agitated
    Severe anemia

A rational approach to thrombolysis and the pharmacologic management of AMI (Fig. 20-1)

- Including hirudin, APSAC, ACE inhibitors, and $MgSO_4$, there are approximately 10 different classes of pharmacologic agents that can be used alone or in combination to treat acute myocardial infarction. This translates into 1023 drug combinations.

Table 20-8 Intravenous heparin monitoring and dosage adjustment

PTT	Rate change (ml/hr)	Dosage change (U/24 hr)	Additional action	Next PTT
< 46	+4	+4800	Rebolus 5000 U	4-6 hr
46-54	+2	+2400	None	4-6 hr
55-80	0	0	None	Next morning
80-110	-2	-2400	Stop infusion 1 hr	4-6 hr after restart
> 110	-4	-4800	Stop infusion 1 hr	4-6 hr after restart

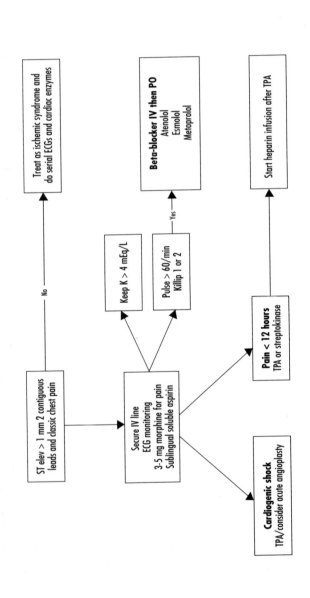

ST elev > 1 mm 2 contiguous leads and classic chest pain

No → Treat as ischemic syndrome and do serial ECGs and cardiac enzymes

Secure IV line
ECG monitoring
3-5 mg morphine for pain
Sublingual soluble aspirin

Keep K > 4 mEq/L

Pulse > 60/min
Killip 1 or 2

Yes →

Beta-blocker IV then PO
Atenolol
Esmolol
Metoprolol

Pain < 12 hours
TPA or streptokinase

Start heparin infusion after TPA

Cardiogenic shock
TPA/consider acute angioplasty

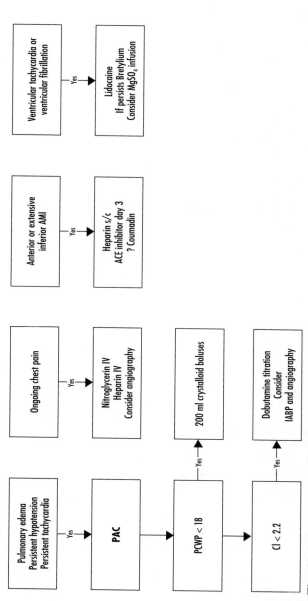

Fig. 20-1 Acute myocardial infarction.

- Unless contraindicated or if the patient has had a "small" infarct, all patients with an acute myocardial infarction who present within 12 hours of the onset of chest pain should receive thrombolytic therapy. t-PA is five to ten times more expensive than streptokinase. *The thrombolytic agent of choice in various clinical scenarios remains unclear.* The results of the thrombolytic megatrials raise two critical questions. First, what is the relative risk-benefit ratio of t-PA compared with SK? Second, what is the cost-effectiveness of t-PA compared with SK?

  In the GUSTO study the combined clinical outcomes of death and nonfatal disabling stroke were 7.7% for SK plus SQ heparin and 6.9% for front-loaded t-PA.

  The GUSTO Economics and Quality-of-Life investigators estimated that the excess cost of t-PA was $21,820 per additional life saved. This is comparable or substantially lower than that of other widely accepted therapies (drug therapy for severe hypertension ($20,000), dialysis ($35,000).

- Patients treated with t-PA should be anticoagulated with heparin. All other patients should receive low-dose SQ heparin.
- All patients should be treated with aspirin, 40 to 175 mg daily (unless the patient has active peptic ulcer disease).
- Unless contraindicated, all patients should be treated with beta-blockers.
- Patients should not be treated with lidocaine (or other antiarrhythmic agents) unless the patient has sustained VT or VF.
- Unless contraindicated, ACE inhibitors should be given, starting on the third to fifth postinfarction day.
- Unless contraindicated, a low-level stress test should be performed before the patient is discharged from hospital.

- Nitroglycerin should not be used unless the patient has postinfarction angina or if thrombolytic agents have not been given.
- Magnesium sulphate should not be given unless the patient is hypomagnesemic.
- Patients at an increased risk of systemic emboli should receive therapeutic doses of heparin followed by warfarin (INR 2.5 to 3.5) for up to 3 months, and then long-term aspirin (warfarin and aspirin should not be given concurrently, except in situations of very high embolic risk). These include patients with the following:

    Anterior q wave infarction
    Severe LV dysfunction
    CHF
    History of systemic or pulmonary emboli
    2D echo evidence of mural thrombus
    Atrial fibrillation (indefinite therapy)

INDICATIONS FOR TEMPORARY PACING IN ACUTE MYOCARDIAL INFARCTION

- Definite
    Asystole
    Complete heart block
- Possible
    RBBB with left anterior or posterior hemiblock developing during acute infarction

    LBBB developing during acute infarction
    LBBB with first-degree heart block of unknown duration

INDICATIONS FOR PULMONARY ARTERY CATHETERIZATION

- Cardiogenic shock
- Severe heart failure

- Suspected mechanical complication
  VSD
  Papillary muscle rupture
  Pericardial tamponade
- Progressive hypotension failing to respond to fluids
- Right ventricular infarction and left ventricular dysfunction

RIGHT VENTRICULAR INFARCTION

Diagnosis

- *Clinical*: a raised JVP, hypotension, and clear chest in a patient with an acute inferior myocardial infarction is characteristic of RV infarction. Kussmaul sign may be positive.
- *Hemodynamic criteria*: RA pressure > 10 mm Hg or a PA/PCWP > 0.8 in a patient with no features of cor pulmonale.
- *ECG criteria*: ST segment elevation in V_{4R}. ST elevation in V_1 with ST depression in V_2 is said to be characteristic of RV infarction.
- *Radionuclide techniques*: these are the most sensitive diagnostic methods, especially MUGA scan or pyrophosphate scan.

Management of RV infarct

- Fluid administration (despite a raised JVP) is the cornerstone of therapy. The optimal CVP is between 10 and 14 mm Hg.
- Patients who have not responded to fluid challenges should have a therapeutic trial of dobutamine. PAC may be useful in these patients.

INDICATIONS (RELATIVE) FOR ACUTE ANGIOGRAPHY AND ANGIOPLASTY IN AMI

- Ongoing chest pain despite maximal medical therapy
- Cardiogenic shock

CHAPTER 21

Tachyarrhythmias

APPROACH TO TACHYARRHYTHMIAS

Refer to Fig. 21-1.

ACUTE ATRIAL FIBRILLATION

Atrial fibrillation (AF) is common in critically ill ICU patients. AF is particularly common in patients with acute pulmonary hypertension (ARDS, pneumonia, etc.) and patients who have undergone cardiac surgery. The management of acute atrial fibrillation in the ICU patient differs significantly from that of the ambulatory patient. AF may cause significant hemodynamic compromise in the critically ill patient. It has been reported that the cardiac output may fall by as much as 30% when the ICU patient develops AF. The management of patients with AF (and flutter) essentially involves the following three steps:

1. Management of precipitating factors (if treatable)
2. Controlling the ventricular response
3. Cardioversion

- Precipitating factors
  Exclude digoxin toxicity
  Hypoxia
  Electrolyte disturbances—hypokalemia, hypocalcemia, hypomagnesemia, hypophosphatemia

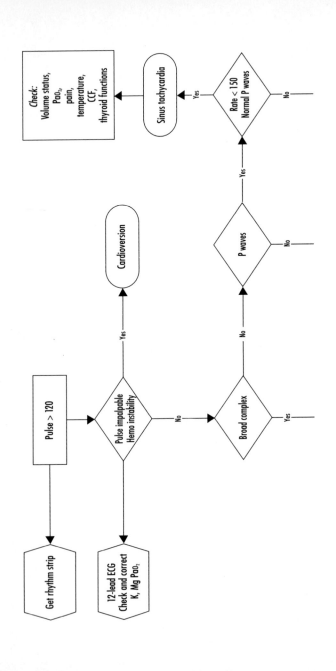

Pulse > 120 → Get rhythm strip

Pulse > 120 → 12-lead ECG Check and correct K, Mg PaO₂

Pulse impalpable Hemo instability — Yes → Cardioversion

Pulse impalpable Hemo instability — No → Broad complex

Broad complex — Yes

Broad complex — No → P waves

P waves — No

P waves — Yes → Rate < 150 Normal P waves

Rate < 150 Normal P waves — Yes → Sinus tachycardia → *Check:* Volume status, PaO₂, pain, temperature, CCF, thyroid functions

Rate < 150 Normal P waves — No

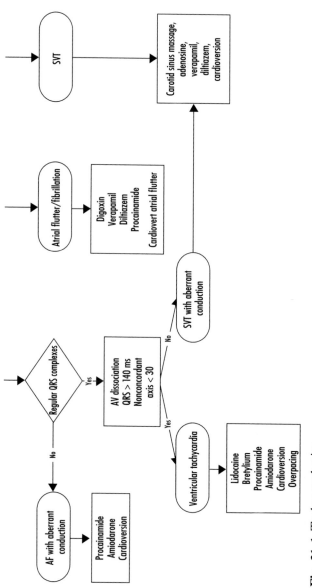

Fig. 21-1 Tachyarrythmias.

Drugs—aminophylline, dopamine, epinephrine, beta-2 agonists

Myocardial ischemia
Pulmonary embolus
Acute increase in pulmonary arterial pressure, worsening ARDS, pulmonary edema

Pericarditis
Hypotension
Hyperthyroidism

- Rate control

  Digoxin (ouabain)

  Loading dose: 0.25 mg repeated 5 minutes later, followed by 0.25 mg q 6 hr for 1 to 3 doses. The usual loading dose is 1 mg/24 hours; the maximal dose is 1.25 mg/24 hours. The loading dose *must* be reduced by approximately 50% in patients with renal failure.

  Maintenance dose: 0.125 to 0.25 mg daily. The maintenance dose *must* be reduced by approximately 50% in patients with renal failure.

  Never give digoxin to a patient with an accessory pathway.

  Beta-blockers: metoprolol, atenolol, or esmolol may be useful if digoxin fails to control the rate.

  Verapamil

  Loading dose: 5 mg over 5 minutes for up to 15 mg
  Maintenance dose: 1 to 5 μ/kg/min
  Verapamil may cause profound hypotension in patients with poor LV function

  Diltiazem

  Loading dose: 5 mg over 3 to 5 minutes up to 15 mg

  Maintenance dose: 2 to 3 μg/kg/min

  Procainamide

  Loading dose: 100 mg until control or 1000 mg, at a rate not to exceed 20 mg/min

  Maintenance dose: 1 to 4 mg/min

- Cardioversion

    Critically ill patients do not tolerate AF well. It may therefore be desirable to attempt cardioversion in the following settings:

    Acute onset

    Hemodynamic compromise

    Angina or postinfarction

This may be achieved either pharmacologically or electrically.

    Procainamide is regarded as the agent of choice. Monitor procainamide and NAPA (major metabolize) levels. The recommended therapeutic concentration of procainamide is 4 to 8 µg/ml, and for NAPA it is 10 to 24 µg/ml, respectively. Daily ECGs to monitor for toxicity; stop drug if QRS duration increases by > 25% or prolonged QTc interval.

    Propafenone (class IC agent) is well tolerated; however, the role of this agent needs to be determined

- *IV Amiodarone* (**not FDA approved**): 5 mg/kg loading dose over 20 minutes, followed by an infusion at 10 mg/kg/24 hours.
- A recent study suggests that parenteral magnesium sulphate may be a useful agent for the treatment of atrial tachyarrhythmias in the ICU (*Crit Care Med* 23:1816, 1995). A bolus of 0.037 g/kg (0.15 mmol/kg) was given over 5 minutes, followed by an infusion at 0.025 g/kg/hr (0.1 mmol/kg/hr). In patients with a serum creatine greater than 3.4 mg/dl or a urine output of less than 40 ml/hr, the infusion rate was reduced to 0.0125 g/kg/hr.

    Synchronized electrical cardioversion: start using low energy (e.g., 30 to 50 J). Digoxin toxicity is a relative contraindication to electrical cardioversion. Low energy and extreme caution should be used when cardioverting any patient taking digoxin. Procainamide is usually required to maintain the patient in sinus after electrical cardioversion.

- Anticoagulation

    It is commonly assumed that left atrial thrombus in patients with atrial fibrillation begins to form after the onset of atrial fibrillation and that it requires greater than 3 days to form. Thus patients with acute atrial fibrillation frequently undergo cardioversion without anticoagulation prophylaxis. However, a recent report demonstrated that a left atrial appendage thrombus was present in 14% of patients with acute (<3 days) atrial fibrillation. In view of this, it may be prudent to anticoagulate all patients with acute atrial fibrillation, unless a contraindication exists.

- ECG manifestations of digoxin toxicity

    Severe sinus bradycardia or junctional rhythm without P waves

    Atrial tachycardia with 2:1 AV block
    First-to-third-degree AV block
    Accelerated idioventricular tachycardia
    Ventricular tachycardia

NOTE:

1. Digoxin is not an antiarrhythmic drug. Digoxin is a proarrhythmic drug. Digoxin will *not* convert a patient from AF to sinus rhythm; it will *not* maintain a patient in sinus rhythm who has been cardioverted from AF; and it has *no* value as a prophylactic agent to prevent AF in ICU patients or post-CABG patients. Digoxin slows the ventricular response (in patient with high adrenergic tone) by increasing vagal tone and slowing AV conduction.

2. Quinidine and disopyramide have no role in the ICU.

CHRONIC ATRIAL FIBRILLATION

Patients with chronic AF are often admitted to the ICU. If the patient has a rapid ventricular response, the drugs already outlined can be used. Digoxin is the drug of choice in a patient with AF and congestive cardiac failure. Beta-blockers are useful in patients with AF and mitral stenosis or hypertension. Unless contraindicated, all patients with AF should be anticoagulated. Aspirin may be used in patients in whom long-term Coumadin is contraindicated. Recent data have shown that patients less than 60 years of age who do not have hypertension, diabetes, valvular heart disease, or ischemic heart disease (lone atrial fibrillation) do not require anticoagulant therapy for stroke prevention because of their low risk (less than 0.5% per year). Patients over the age of 60 years with lone atrial fibrillation seem to be adequately protected with aspirin.

Should AF be of recent onset (less than 1 year), and echocardiography demonstrates left atrium less than 4.5 cm in diameter, cardioversion can be attempted. This may be achieved pharmacologically or electrically. Low-dose amiodarone (100 to 200 mg/day) is currently considered the drug of choice to achieve and maintain sinus rhythm. However, the patient must be anticoagulated before cardioversion and for at least 2 weeks after successful cardioversion.

Regimen for chronic anticoagulation includes the following:

- Control the blood pressure to reduce the risk of intracerebral bleeding.
- Monitor using INR. Data from *The European Atrial Fibrillation Trial* suggest that the INR should be kept between 2.0 and 4.0, with a target INR of 3.0.
- Age < 70: start 4 mg Coumadin per day
  Age > 70: start 3 mg Coumadin per day
- If INR > 4.0, reduce by 1 mg
  If INR < 2, increase by 1 mg

ATRIAL FLUTTER

Atrial flutter is usually associated with underlying heart disease. It is important to identify and treat any underlying cause. It is usually very difficult to slow the ventricular response below 150 beats/min with the use of AV nodal blocking drugs. The persistent administration of drugs such as digoxin or verapamil usually results in toxicity before the ventricular response is controlled. The preferred method of control is electrical cardioversion. This can usually be achieved with low energy, 20 to 50 J. Atrial flutter can also be converted to sinus rhythm by overdrive atrial pacing.

PAROXYSMAL SUPRAVENTRICULAR TACHYCARDIA (PSVT)

Atrioventricular nodal reentrant tachycardia is usually not associated with underlying heart disease and may be precipitated by the same factors as atrial fibrillation or atrial flutter. This arrhythmia is characterized by a sudden onset and sudden termination. The rate may range from 150 to 200 beats/min but most often is 180 to 200 beats/min. Because there is almost simultaneous excitation of both the atria and ventricles, the P wave occurs at the time of the QRS complex and is difficult to appreciate on the electrocardiogram.

Management

- Vagal maneuvers are the initial treatment of choice
    Valsalva maneuver
    Müller maneuver—deep inspiration against a closed glottis

    Carotid sinus massage—check that the patient has no carotid bruit or history of TIAs
- Electrical cardioversion if the patient is hemodynamically unstable; 100 to 200 J
- Adenosine is the pharmacologic agent of choice in patients who have failed vagal maneuvers. The usual dose is 6 to 12 mg by slow IV push. After termination of the tachycardia, brief periods of asystole are common.
- Verapamil is also effective in terminating a PSVT.

- Because of denervation-hypersensitivity, adenosine should not be given to heart transplant recipients.

WOLFF-PARKINSON-WHITE (WPW) SYNDROME

The following acute therapies are available for an orthodromic reciprocating tachycardia (Table 21-1).
- Electrical cardioversion if the patient is hemodynamically unstable
- Adenosine is the pharmacologic agent of choice (6 to 12 mg IV)
- Procainamide may be safely used in WPW syndrome
- *Digoxin and verapamil should not be administered* because they can shorten the refractory period of the bypass tract.
- Adenosine, digoxin, and calcium channel blockers should *not* be given to patients who have atrial fibrillation with an accessory pathway because blocking AV nodal conduction may provoke conduction down the accessory pathway, leading to an increase in the ventricular rate and hemodynamic collapse. The treatment of choice for these patients is procainamide.

Table 21-1 Long-term antiarrhythmic drug treatment of supraventricular tachycardias

Tachycardia	First choice	Second choice
AV nodal reentrant	Calcium-channel blockers, Beta-blockers	Flecainide, propafenone
WPW syndrome	Flecainide, propafenone, quinidine, procainamide	Beta-blockers

ACCELERATED IDIOVENTRICULAR RHYTHM

Accelerated idioventricular rhythm is characterized by a wide QRS complex and a regular ventricular rate, usually 60 to 110 beats/min. This is a benign rhythm that is usually asymptomatic and should just be observed.

VENTRICULAR PREMATURE COMPLEXES AND BIGEMINY

These are recognized by wide QRS complexes (> 120 ms) with a bizarre configuration. Identify and treat possible precipitating factors, such as hypoxia and electrolyte disturbances. Ensure that the K^+ > 4 mEq/L and that the Mg^{2+} > 2 mg/dl. Treat the underlying cause and *not* the VPCs.

Frequent VPCs (> 6/min), multifocal VPCs, couplets, and R on T VPCs occurring within the first 6 hours of an acute myocardial infarction are often treated with lidocaine. This arrhythmia increases the patient's risk; however, there are no strong data to indicate that suppression of these PVCs reduces the incidence of ventricular fibrillation or impacts on patient outcome. During the later hospital phase, frequent VPCs (more than 10/h, multifocal beats, or couplets) may increase risk, but there are limited data that antiarrhythmic therapy, other than beta-blocking agents alters patient outcome. The Cardiac Arrhythmia Suppression Trial (CAST) indicated an increase in mortality among these patients with the use of flecainide and encainide. These patients should be treated with a beta-blocking agent such as metoprolol (should no contraindication exist to the use of this class of drugs).

NONSUSTAINED VENTRICULAR TACHYCARDIA

Nonsustained ventricular tachycardia is defined as three consecutive PVCs up to 30 seconds at a rate of > 100 beats/min. This arrhythmia is usually associated with underlying heart disease and is associated with an increased mortality. In the ICU setting precipitating factors should be diagnosed and treated. In the setting of acute myocardial ischemia progressively longer runs of this arrhythmia may herald the onset of VF and should therefore be suppressed. In most other situations, unless the patient is symptomatic, this arrhythmia should be observed.

SUSTAINED VENTRICULAR TACHYCARDIA

Is a wide QRS complex tachycardia ectopy or aberration?

- Factors favoring ectopy
    AV dissociation
    R or qR in V_1 with taller *left* rabbit ear
    QS or RS in V_6
    Bizarre frontal plane axis
    Concordant V leads
    LBBB pattern with wide r in V_1
- Factors favoring SVT with aberration
    Preceding P wave
    RBBB pattern
    Triphasic contour in V_1 and V_6
    Initial vector identical to that of flanking conducted beats

    qRs in V_6

If there is any doubt, the arrhythmia should be considered to be ventricular rather than supraventricular. Adenosine may be used to differentiate between these two arrhythmias. The treatment of a ventricular tachycardia with verapamil can result in a fatal outcome.

Sustained ventricular tachycardia usually occurs in patients with severe underlying heart disease, usually ischemic heart disease. The prognosis depends largely on that of the underlying heart disease. The treatment of patients with sustained VT is dependent on the hemodynamic consequences. Cardioversion is the treatment of choice in hemodynamically compromised patients. If the patient is asymptomatic or only mildly symptomatic, a number of the therapeutic options can be pursued (alone and in combination) including the following:

- Elective synchronized cardioversion
- Procainamide is considered the drug of choice. Loading dose of 15 mg/kg at rate of 25 to 50 mg/min followed by an infusion at 1 to 4 mg/min. Monitor levels and ECG as described previously.
- *Amiodarone*: IV (***not yet FDA approved***) or high-dose oral loading
- Implantable antitachycardia device
- *Sotalol*: PO 80 to 320 mg/day; avoid with concurrent diuretic use (torsades de pointes)

SUSTAINED VENTRICULAR TACHYCARDIA IN THE SETTING OF ACUTE ISCHEMIA

- Treat underlying ischemia
- *Lidocaine*: 1 mg/kg LD, followed by 0.5 mg/kg in 20 minutes, infusion of 1 to 4 mg/min
- Beta-blocking agent
- *Bretylium*: 5 to 10 mg/kg LD, followed by infusion of 0.5 to 4 mg/min
- *Amiodarone*: IV (***not yet FDA approved***) or high-dose oral loading

POLYMORPHIC VENTRICULAR TACHYCARDIA (TORSADES DE POINTES)

The hallmark of polymorphic ventricular tachycardia (PVT) is a QRS morphology that changes constantly. Torsades de pointes translated means "twisting of the points." Multiple leads may be required to demonstrate this phenomenon. This arrhythmia is classified as being associated with either a normal QT interval or a prolonged QT interval.

- Normal QT interval
    Acute myocardial ischemia
    Hypertrophic cardiomyopathy
    Dilated cardiomyopathy
- Prolonged QT interval
    Congenital long QT syndrome
    Acute myocardial ischemia
    Antiarrhythmic drugs, especially class I agents; rarely sotalol (hypokalemia) and amiodarone

    Other drugs, including phenothiazines, tricyclic antidepressants, erythromycin, ampicillin, pentamidine

    Electrolyte disturbances
      Hypokalemia
      Hypomagnesemia
      Hypocalcemia
    Acute intracranial pathology, such as subarachnoid hemorrhage and intracerebral bleeding
- Management
    Electrolyte abnormalities must be aggressively corrected, particularly potassium and magnesium deficiency.

    Magnesium sulphate (1 to 2 g) is usually highly successful, even in the absence of magnesium deficiency. 2 g (10 ml of 20% solution) is given IV over 10 minutes, followed by 4 g over 4 to 8 hours as an infusion.

    Accelerating the heart rate is a simple and quick method of shortening the QT interval. Transvenous pacing is a safe and effective method of controlling this arrhythmia. As an immediate measure transcutaneous pacing may be used while preparations are being made for electrode placement.

    An infusion of isoproterenol (2 to 8 µg/min) titrated to increase the heart rate above 120 beats/min is sometimes used if pacing is not available. Isoproterenol is contraindicated in patients with an acute myocardial infarction, active ischemia, and severe hypertension.

If the arrhythmia occurs during therapy with a type 1A agent, amiodarone may terminate the arrhythmia.

PVT occurring in the setting of myocardial ischemia does not usually respond to antiarrhythmic therapy. These patients usually require coronary revascularization. If the QT interval is prolonged, standard class I antiarrhythmic agents should not be used.

Patients with the congenital long QT syndrome are usually treated with beta-blockers or phenytoin.

CHAPTER 22

Bradyarrhythmias

SINUS BRADYCARDIA

Sinus bradycardia is not uncommon in ICU patients. This may occur because of myocardial ischemia, digoxin toxicity, sick sinus syndrome, or beta-blockers and calcium channel blockers. The patient should *only* be treated if symptomatic.

- Atropine 0.5 mg repeated up to total of 3 mg
- Isoproterenol 1 to 2 µg/min up to 20 µg/min
- A dopamine infusion, especially in hypotensive patients
- Pacing
    Transvenous temporary pacemaker
    External pacemaker (transcutaneous)

SICK SINUS SYNDROME

Sick sinus syndrome is also known as the *tachycardia-bradycardia syndrome*. As the name implies these patients have episodes of both tachycardia and bradycardia. The critically ill patient with this syndrome often requires temporary pacing to achieve hemodynamic stability.

CHAPTER **23** _____

Pacing

INDICATIONS FOR TEMPORARY PACING

- In the setting of acute myocardial infarction
  Asystole
  Complete heart block
  ? *New* RBBB *and new* LAH or LPH (i.e., new bifascicular block)
  ? New left bundle branch block
  Symptomatic bradycardia not responsive to atropine
- Other settings
  Overdrive pacing
  Symptomatic bradycardia not responsive to atropine (e.g., beta-blocker OD)

  An ICU patient with the tachy-brady syndrome (sick sinus syndrome)
  Prophylaxis before surgery
    Patients with a bifascicular block and a history of syncope

    Patients with bifascicular block and AV nodal disease

Pacemaker codes (Table 23-1)

The following pacing modes are currently used in different clinical situations:

VVI: demand ventricular pacing; output inhibited by sensed ventricular signals

Table 23-1 Pacemaker codes

Chamber paced	Chamber sensed	Response to sensing	Programmability	Antitachycardiac functions
O	O	O	O	O
A	A	I	S†	P
V	V	T	M	S‡
D	D	D	C	D
			R	

O, None; A, atrium; I, inhibited; S†, simple; P, antitachycardia; V, ventricle; T, triggered; M, multiprogrammable; S‡, shock; D, dual; C, communicating; R, rate modulation.

AAI: demand atrial pacing; output inhibited by sensed ventricular signals

DDI: VVI plus AAI pacing, tracking of atrial rate by ventricular sensing does not occur

DDD: paces and senses both atrium and ventricles; synchronizes with atrial activity and paces ventricle after present AV interval

DDDR: DDD pacing with sensor-based increase or decrease in paced atrial and ventricular rates in response to changes in metabolic demand

VVIR: VVI pacing with sensor-based changes in pacing rates based on metabolic demand

AAIR: AAI pacing with variable atrial pacing rate based on changes in metabolic demand

VOO: fixed rate (asynchronous) ventricular pacing

AAT: triggered atrial pacing; output pulse delivered into P waves; paces atrium at a preset interval

VVT: triggered ventricular pacing; output pulse delivered into R waves; paces ventricle at a preset escape interval

AAO: fixed rate (synchronous) atrial pacing

DVI: pacing in atrium and ventricle; senses R wave only

VDD: paces in ventricle; senses both atrium and ventricle; synchronizes with atrial activity and paces ventricle after a preset AV interval

PART THREE

METABOLIC AND ENDOCRINE PROBLEMS IN THE ICU

Acid-base disturbances

BLOOD GAS INTERPRETATION

Refer to Tables 24-1 to 24-4.

AN APPROACH TO BLOOD GAS DETERMINATION

Task 1: Is there an acid-base disorder?

Look at the Pa_{CO_2} and the HCO_3 to determine whether they are in the normal range (Table 24-1). If they are abnormal, go to task 2; if they are normal, go to task 5.

Task 2: Is the patient acidemic or alkalemic?

Look at the pH. If the pH is normal (i.e., between 7.35 and 7.45), is the pH on the acidemic or alkalemic side of 7.40?

Table 24-1 Normal acid-base ranges

Variable	Mean	1 SD	2 SD
Pa_{CO_2} (mm Hg)	40	38-42	35-45
pH	7.40	7.38-7.42	7.35-7.45
HCO_3	24	23-25	22-26

Table 24-2 Acid-base terminology

Clinical terminology	Criteria
Respiratory failure/respiratory acidosis	$Pa_{CO_2} > 45$ mm Hg
Alveolar hyperventilation (respiratory alkalosis)	$Pa_{CO_2} < 35$ mm Hg
Acute respiratory failure	$Pa_{CO_2} > 45$ mm Hg; pH < 7.35
Chronic respiratory failure	$Pa_{CO_2} > 45$ mm Hg; pH 7.36-7.44
Acute respiratory alkalosis	$Pa_{CO_2} < 35$ mm Hg; pH > 7.45
Chronic respiratory alkalosis	$Pa_{CO_2} < 35$ mm Hg; pH 7.36-7.44
Acidemia	pH < 7.35
Alkalemia	pH > 7.45
Acidosis	$HCO_3 < 22$ mEq/L
Alkalosis	$HCO_3 > 26$ mEq/L

Task 3: What is the primary acid-base disorder?

From an analysis of the pH, Pa_{CO_2}, and HCO_3, determine the primary metabolic defect.

I.   If the pH is decreased, the patient has an acidemia, which may be either of the following:
   A.   Metabolic acidosis, which is characterized by a low HCO_3
   B.   Respiratory acidosis, which is characterized by an increased P_{CO_2}

II. If the pH is increased, the patient has an alkalemia, which may be either of the following:
   A.   Metabolic alkalosis, which is characterized by an increase in plasma HCO_3
   B.   Respiratory alkalosis, which is characterized by a decreased P_{CO_2}

Table 24-3 Traditional acid-base definitions

Disorder and definition	Compensatory response	pH	PaCO$_2$	HCO$_3$	BE
Respiratory acidosis (defined as increased PaCO$_2$)	Uncompensated	↓	↑	N	N
	Partly compensated	↓	↑	↑	↑
	Compensated	N	↑	↑	↑
Respiratory alkalosis (defined as decreased PaCO$_2$)	Uncompensated	↑	↓	N	N
	Partly compensated	↑	↓	↓	↓
	Compensated	N	↓	↓	↓
Metabolic acidosis (defined as decreased HCO$_3$)	Uncompensated	↓	N	↓	↓
	Partly compensated	↓	↓	↓	↓
	Compensated	N	↓	↓	↓
Metabolic alkalosis (defined as decreased HCO$_3$)	Uncompensated	↑	N	↑	↑
	Partly compensated	↑	↑	↑	↑
	Compensated	N	↑	↑	↑

Table 24-4 Compensation for acid-base disorders

Primary disorder	Primary change	Compensatory change	Expected compensation
Metabolic acidosis	$\downarrow HCO_3$	$\downarrow PaCO_2$	$\Delta PaCO_2 = 1.2\ \Delta HCO_3$
Metabolic alkalosis	$\uparrow HCO_3$	$\uparrow PaCO_2$	$\Delta PaCO_2 = 0.8\ \Delta HCO_3$
Respiratory acidosis	$\uparrow PaCO_2$	$\uparrow HCO_3$	Acute: $\Delta HCO_3 = 0.1\ \Delta PaCO_2$
			Chronic: $\Delta HCO_3 = 0.35\ \Delta PaCO_2$
Respiratory alkalosis	$\downarrow PaCO_2$	$\downarrow HCO_3$	Acute: $\Delta HCO_3 = 0.2\ \Delta PaCO_2$
			Chronic: $\Delta HCO_3 = 0.5\ \Delta PaCO_2$

Task 4: Expected compensatory response

Determine whether the compensatory response is of the magnitude expected (Tables 24-3 and 24-4), i.e., is there a secondary (uncompensated) acid-base disturbance?

Task 5: How to recognize mixed acid-base disorders

Acid-base disorders may present as two or three co-existing disorders. It is possible for a patient to have an acid-base disorder with a normal pH, P_{CO_2}, and HCO_3, with the only clue to an acid-base disorder being an increased anion gap.

Anion Gap = [Na] − ([Cl] + [HCO_3]): Normal 12 ± 2 mEq/L

I.   Calculate the plasma anion gap; if it is increased by > 5 mEq/L, the patient most likely has a *metabolic acidosis*.

II. Compare the fall in plasma HCO_3 (25 − HCO_3) with the increase in the plasma anion gap; these should be of similar magnitude. If there is a gross discrepancy (5 mEq/L), there is a mixed disturbance present.
    A. If increase AG < fall HCO_3, suggests that a component of the metabolic acidosis is caused by HCO_3 loss
    B. If increase AG > fall HCO_3, sugests coexistent metabolic alkalosis

Task 6: Calculate the osmolar gap

Calculate the osmolar gap in patients with an unexplained AG metabolic acidosis (Table 24-5).

Estimated serum osmolality = 2 × Na + glucose/18 + BUN/2.8

$$Normal \approx 290 \ mosm/kg.H_2O$$

Osmolal gap = osm (measured) − osm (calculated); normal < 10

Table 24-5 Osmolal gap and lethal intoxications

Substance	Mol wt	Lethal level (mg/dl)	Osm gap at that level
Ethanol	46	350	80
Isopropyl alcohol	60	340	60
Methanol	32	80	27
Acetone	58	55	10
Ethylene glycol	62	21	4

Causes of an increased osmolal gap

- Alcohol (ethanol)
- Methanol
- Isopropyl alcohol (does not cause an anion gap or an acidosis)
- Ethylene glycol
- Mannitol
- Sorbitol
- Paraldehyde
- Acetone

Some further thoughts on acid-base disturbances

I. Only a metabolic acidosis caused by $NaHCO_3$ loss leads to an initial hyperkalemia (H^+ ions enter the cell and are buffered in the ICF; K^+ leaves the cell to maintain electrical neutrality). In contrast, a gain of organic acid does not cause initial hyperkalemia. With organic acid loads, the organic anions ($lactate^-$, beta-hydroxybutyrate$^-$) enter the ICF in close to equal quantity to that of H^+. Thus, little K^+ shift is required for electrical neutrality. K^+ shifts into the ICF in metabolic alkalosis.

II. Respiratory acid-base disorders cause minimal changes in plasma K^+.

III. *D-lactic acidosis*: certain bacteria in the GI tract may convert carbohydrate into organic acids. The two factors that make this possible are slow GI transit (blind loops, obstruction) and change of the normal flora (usually with antibiotic therapy). The most prevalent organic acid is D-lactic acid. Since humans metabolize this isomer more slowly than L-lactate, and production rates can be very rapid, life-threatening acidosis can be produced. This usual laboratory test for lactate is specific for the L-lactate isomer. Therefore to confirm the diagnosis, the plasma D-lactate must be measured.

Useful acid-base formula

$$H_2CO_3 = P_{CO_2} \times 0.03 \text{ (Normal = 1.3 mEq/L)}$$

$$TCO_2 = HCO_3 + H_2CO_3$$

$$pH \approx HCO_3 / H_2CO_3 \text{ (20:1 at pH of 7.4)}$$

METABOLIC ALKALOSIS

Refer to Fig. 24-1.

METABOLIC ACIDOSIS

Refer to Fig. 24-2.

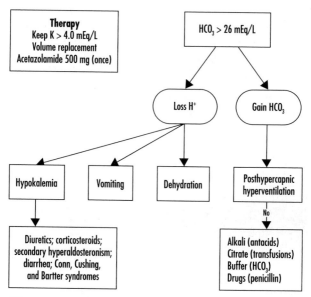

Fig. 24-1 Metabolic alkalosis.

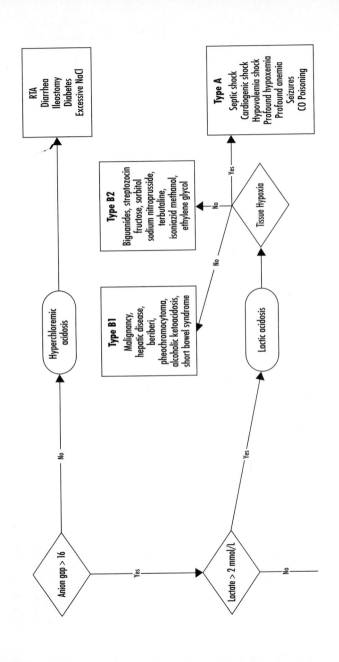

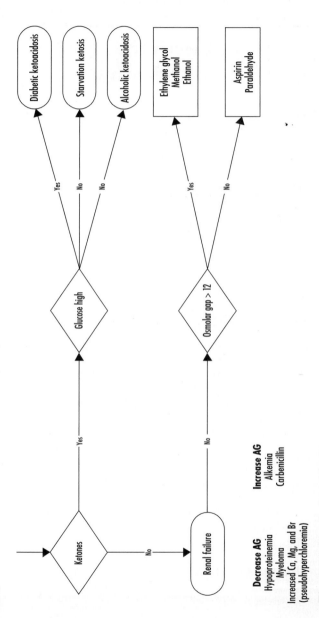

Fig. 24-2 Metabolic acidosis.

CHAPTER 25

Electrolyte disturbances

RULES

- Water (without Na^+) crosses the cell membrane until the osmolality is equal on both sides of that membrane. Water balance determines tonicity and not ECF volume.

    Increased total body water (only) causes hyponatremia but not edema

    Decreased total body water (only) causes hypernatremia but not dehydration
- Intracellular fluid (ICF) particles rarely change
- *Na^+ content = ECF volume*: body Na content determines the ECF volume, and the ECF (Na) reflects the ICF volume

    Patients who are dehydrated have a low total body Na^+, regardless of the serum Na^+ concentration

    Patients who have edema (increased ECF volume) have an increased total body Na+, regardless of the serum Na+ concentration
- No body fluid has a higher osmolarity (or Na^+ concentration) than plasma

HYPONATREMIA

Refer to Fig. 25-1.

HYPOKALEMIA

Diagnostic approach

Refer to Fig. 25-2.

Replacement of K+

- Only a fraction of the total body K^+ is extracellular. Therefore serum K^+ levels do not accurately reflect the total body K^+. The degree of K^+ deficit is dependent on the duration of the precipitating cause (time for equilibration) and the serum K^+ level. In patients with chronic hypokalemia, a 1 mEq fall in serum K^+ is approximately equal to a 200 mEq total body deficit.
- Check and correct phosphate and magnesium levels.

IV replacement therapy of KCl

- No more than 20 mEq/hr should be given
- Central line infusion
  - 20 mEq in 50 ml over 1 hour
  - 40 mEq in 100 ml over 2 hours
- Peripheral line infusion
  - 10 mEq in 100 ml over 1 hour
  - 20 mEq in 200 ml over 2 hours

HYPERKALEMIA

- Clinical features usually occur when the $K^+ > 6.5$ mEq/L: weakness, paresthesia, ileus, paralysis, cardiac arrest
- ECG changes
  - Peaked T waves
  - Flattened P waves
  - Prolonged PR interval
  - Widening of the QRS complex
  - Sine wave leading to ventricular fibrillation or asystole

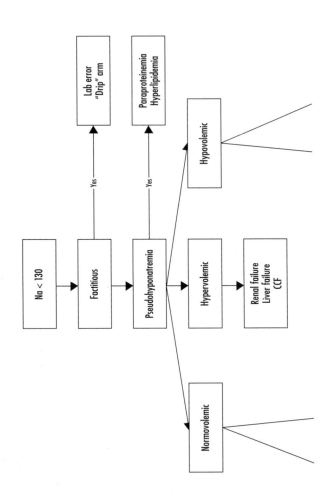

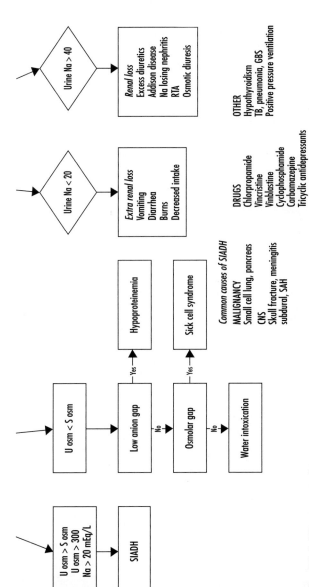

Fig. 25-1 Hyponatremia.

U osm > S osm
U osm > 300
Na > 20 mEq/L → SIADH

U osm < S osm → Low anion gap —Yes→ Hypoproteinemia

Low anion gap —No→ Osmolar gap —Yes→ Sick cell syndrome

Osmolar gap —No→ Water intoxication

Urine Na < 20 → *Extra renal loss*
Vomiting
Diarrhea
Burns
Decreased intake

Urine Na > 40 → *Renal loss*
Excess diuretics
Addison disease
Na losing nephritis
RTA
Osmotic diuresis

Common causes of SIADH
MALIGNANCY
Small cell lung, pancreas
CNS
Skull fracture, meningitis
subdural, SAH

DRUGS
Chlorpropamide
Vincristine
Vinblastine
Cyclophosphamide
Carbamazepine
Tricyclic antidepressants

OTHER
Hypothyroidism
TB, pneumonia, GBS
Positive pressure ventilation

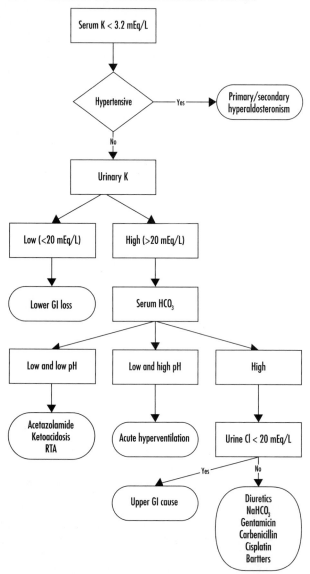

Fig. 25-2 Hypokalemia.

- The rate of progression of the ECG changes is not predictable, and patients may progress from minor ECG changes to dangerous conduction disturbances or arrhythmias within minutes. The ECG changes are exacerbated by coexisting hyponatremia, hypocalcemia, hypermagnesemia, and acidosis.
- Patients should be treated when the K^+ is greater than 5.5 mEq/L: urgent treatment is required when the K^+ > 7.0 mEq/L.
- The goals of treatment are the following:

    Protect the heart from the effects of K^+ by antagonizing the effect on cardiac conduction (calcium)

    Shift the K^+ from the extracellular to the intracellular compartment

    Reduce the total body potassium

- Life-threatening arrhythmia may occur at any time during therapy; hence, continuous ECG monitoring is required.
- Patients with a serum K^+ > 7 mEq/L and/or significant ECG changes should be treated immediately with calcium gluconate, followed by a glucose-insulin infusion and then an iron exchange resin (Table 25-1).

HYPOPHOSPHATEMIA

Phosphorus is an essential component of phospholipids and nucleic acids and plays an essential role in energy metabolism. Only about 1% of the total body phosphorus is extracellular, with the major phosphate store being in bone and the intracellular compartment. The normal range of serum phosphorus concentration in the serum is between 2.2 and 4.4 mg/dl, of which about 55% is in an ionized form that is physiologically active. The serum phosphate concentration is a poor indicator of the total body phosphorus, and rapid shifts of phosphate between the extracellular and intracellular compartments only confound this situation. Interpretation of the serum phosphate

Table 25-1 Agents used in the treatment of hyperkalemia

Agent	Mechanism	Dosage	Onset of action
10% Ca gluconate	Direct antagonism	10-20 ml IV over 2-5 min	Immediate
Sodium bicarbonate	Redistribution	50 ml IV over 2-5 min	Minutes
Glucose-insulin	Redistribution	2-3 g glucose/U regular insulin 50 ml 50% DW + 10 U insulin	Minutes
Sodium polystyrene sulphonate (Kayexalate)	Increased elimination	15-60 g PO or rectally	2-12 hr

is further complicated by a normal diurnal variation, which may be as large as 0.5 mg/dl. However, hypophosphatemia may cause severe, life-threatening complications, particularly in patients with depleted phosphate stores.

- Causes of severe hypophosphatemia
    - Alcohol abuse and withdrawal
    - Refeeding after starvation
    - Respiratory alkalosis
    - Malabsorption
    - Oral phosphate binders
    - Hyperalimentation
    - Severe burns
    - Therapy of diabetic ketoacidosis

There is a poor correlation between serum phosphate levels and symptoms. Although hypophosphatemia becomes life threatening when the serum levels are less than 1 mg/dl, symptoms may develop when the serum phosphate is less than 2 mg/dl.

- Manifestations of hypophosphatemia include the following:
    - Myocardial depression
    - Weakness, rhabdomyolysis, and respiratory failure
    - Confusion, stupor, coma, seizures
    - Hemolysis, platelet dysfunction, leukocyte dysfunction
- Management
    - Therapy is usually empiric, and levels must be closely followed to prevent hyperphosphatemia.

    It has been recommended that patients with severe hypophosphatemia (serum phosphate level less than 1 mg/dl) be given an infusion of phosphate at a rate of 6 mg/kg/hr (or 0.1 mM phosphate/kg in 500 ml 0.45 NS over 6 hours), with serum levels being checked every 6 hours and discontinued when the serum phosphate level exceeds 2 mg/dl. Thereafter the patients should receive oral phosphate to replace the intracellular stores. Phosphate solutions should be used with extreme caution in patients with renal failure. Patients with mild to moderate hypophosphatemia (serum phosphate between 1.0 and 2.2 mg/dl) should receive oral supplementation (1 g Neutra-Phos/day) unless diarrhea precludes using this route of supplementation.

HYPOMAGNESEMIA

- Causes
  - Alcoholism and alcohol withdrawal
  - Decreased intestinal absorption
  - Hypercalcemia
  - Drugs
    - Loop diuretics
    - Aminoglycosides
    - Amphotericin B
    - Cisplatin
    - Cyclosporine
- Manifestations
  - Hypomagnesemia causes hypokalemia and hypocalcemia, which contributes to the clinical picture
  - Lethargy, confusion, coma, seizures, ataxia, nystagmus
  - Prolonged PR and QT intervals on ECG
  - Atrial and ventricular arrhythmias
- Management
  - Severe hypomagnesemia should be treated with 50% magnesium sulphate (4 mEq/ml), 2 to 4 ml IV over 15 minutes, followed by 32 mEq in 1 or more liters of IV fluid over 24 hours.

HYPERCALCEMIA (Table 25-2)

Causes

- Malignancy
  - Lung
  - Breast

Table 25-2 Treatment of hypercalcemia

Agent	Dose	Indication/toxicity
Normal saline	200–400 ml/hr	First line therapy; especially for dehydration
Furosemide	10–40 mg IV q 4–6 hr	Once patient is rehydrated
Etidronate	7.5 mg/kg/day IV; up to 7 days	Avoid in renal failure
Pamidronate	Single dose 60–90 mg over 24 hr (can be given over 4 hr)	Avoid in renal failure
Mithramycin	25 μg/kg IV	Bone marrow suppression
Calcitonin	2–8 IU/kg IM q 6 hr	Acts rapidly; effect not complete and wears off rapidly
Steroids—prednisone	40–100 mg/day	Hematologic malignancies, breast cancer

  Multiple myeloma
  Lymphoma, other
• Primary hyperparathyroidism
• Immobilization
• Drugs
  Thiazides
  Lithium
  Theophylline, other
• Granulomatous diseases
  Sarcoid
  Tuberculosis
• Hypervitaminosis A and D
• Hyperthyroidism
• Milk-alkali syndrome

HYPOCALCEMIA

Hypocalcemia (ionized calcium < 1 mmol/L or 4 mg/dl) is a frequent finding in critically ill patients. Many factors interact to lower the serum calcium. Furthermore, critically ill patients have an impaired ability to mobilize skeletal calcium because of parathormone or vitamin D deficiency.

Cardiovascular manifestations are the most commonly encountered features of hypocalcemia seen in critically ill patients. Patients may develop hypotension, decreased cardiac output, bradycardia, and arrhythmias. In addition, patients may fail to respond to drugs that act through calcium-regulated mechanisms (digoxin, catecholamines). It is important to note that mild degrees of hypocalcemia (ionized calcium > 0.8 mmol/L) are rarely associated with cardiovascular compromise.

Serum ionized calcium should be routinely monitored in critically ill patients, and treatment is recommended when the ionized calcium concentration is below 0.8 mmol/L. The serum magnesium and phosphorus levels should be measured and corrected.

A large body of evidence suggests that cellular calcium overload contributes to cellular dysfunction and death in patients with tissue ischemia. Critically ill patients may have increased intracellular free calcium concentrations, even when the circulating ionized calcium is low. Administration of calcium to these patients may be detrimental by activating autolytic intracellular enzymes. Thus calcium should only be given after confirmation of ionized hypocalcemia to prevent further tissue damage.

Hypocalcemia is a common complication of rhabdomyolysis. Release of phosphate from injured muscle results in the local precipitation of calcium salts. Hyperphosphatemia also impairs the 1-hydroxylation of vitamin D, thereby decreasing the sensitivity of bone to parathormone. Administration of calcium may result in severe soft tissue calcification. Calcium supplementation should be reserved for patients with clear clinical signs of hypocalcemia.

CHAPTER 26

Diabetes mellitus

MANAGEMENT OF DIABETIC KETOACIDOSIS

Refer to Table 26-1 and Fig. 26-1.

In ketoacidosis, the two ketoacids beta-hydroxybutyrate and acetoacetate are in equilibrium.

Acetoacetate + NADH $\leftrightarrows$ Beta-hydroxybutyrate + NAD

The nitroprusside qualitative side room test for ketones detects acetoacetate and acetone only. Therefore if one had NADH accumulation in the mitochondrion, such as in lactic acidosis or in alcohol metabolism, it displaces the equilibrium to the right in favor of beta-hydroxybutyrate. Since the nitroprusside test does not detect beta-hydroxybutyrate, the results may well be only weakly positive, and one may underestimate the ketosis. However, the enzymatic assay for beta-hydroxybutyrate is reliable.

Corrected Na

Corrected Na^+ = 0.016 (measured glucose − 100) + measured Na^+

Severe hyperglycemia

Severe hyperglycemia (glucose > 1000 mg/dl occurs in the following two situations:

Table 26-1 Laboratory values in DKA and hyperosmolar nonketotic coma (HNKC)

Lab test	DKA	HNKC
Blood glucose (mg/dl)	200–2000	Usually > 600
Blood ketones (beta-hydroxybutyrate)	Present (may be absent initially because of acetoacetate)	Absent
Arterial pH	< 7.35	Normal (may be low with severe dehydration and lactic acidosis)
Anion gap	> 18	Normal (or elevated)
Osmolarity	Slightly increased	Elevated
Urine dipstick	Ketones + glucose	Glucose
BUN	Mild to moderate increase	May be markedly increased
Age	Usually young, type I diabetic	Usually elderly

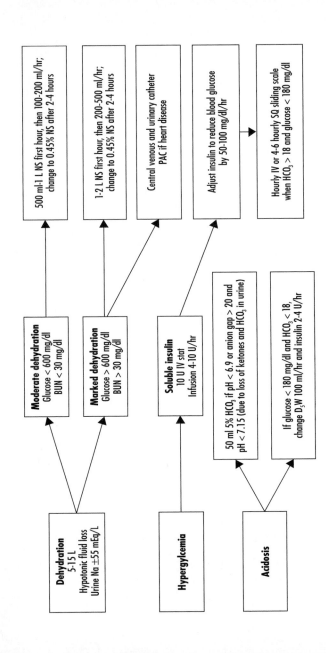

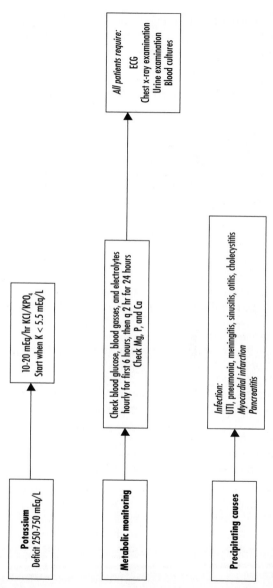

Potassium

Deficit 250-750 mEq/L

10-20 mEq/hr KCl/KPO$_4$

Start when K < 5.5 mEq/L

Metabolic monitoring

Check blood glucose, blood gasses, and electrolytes hourly for first 6 hours, then q 2 hr for 24 hours

Check Mg, P, and Ca

Precipitating causes

Infection:

UTI, pneumonia, meningitis, sinusitis, otitis, cholecystitis

Myocardial infarction

Pancreatitis

All patients require:

ECG

Chest x-ray examination

Urine examination

Blood cultures

Fig. 26-1 Diabetic ketoacidosis.

- Severe dehydration
- Chronic renal failure with low GFR and diminished excretion of glucose (GFR < 25% normal with blood glucose of ± 1000 mg/dl)

Insulin drip protocol for DKA (for BS > 350 mg/dl)

- Mix 50 U in 50 ml NS or 100 U in 100 ml NS (1 U/ml)
- Bolus 10 U
- Infusion 0.1 U/kg/hr

  Monitor fingertip blood glucose q hour and serum glucose, potassium, and blood gasses (arterial or venous) q 2 to 4 hours until glucose is stable

  If blood sugar (BS) does not decrease by 100 mg/dl within 2 hours, double the infusion rate (repeat as required)

  Once BS < 250 mg/dl, halve infusion rate, and add D_5W

  Titrate infusion (as outlined below) until the HCO_3 > 18 mEq/L. Then change to a 4 to 6 hourly SQ sliding scale (for DKA)
- Hourly insulin titration

  BS 201 to 300: increase infusion by 1 U/hr until BS decreases to < 200

  BS 121 to 200: do not change infusion rate

  BS 90 to 120: decrease infusion to 1 U/hr

  BS < 90: stop infusion; start at 1 U/hr when BS > 200

Insulin regimen for management of the hyperglycemic patient in the ICU

- Mix 50 U in 50 ml NS or 100 U in 100 ml NS (1 U/ml)
- Bolus

  Blood glucose < 250 mg/dl—no bolus

  Blood glucose > 250 mg/dl—2-unit bolus

  Blood glucose > 300 mg/dl—5-unit bolus
- Start infusion at 3 U/hr

- Monitor fingertip blood glucose hourly, and serum glucose and potassium every 4 to 6 hours until glucose is stable
- Hourly insulin titration

  BS > 300:   increase infusion by 2 U/hr until BS < 300 (increase infusion by 3 U/hr if BS is declining at a rate less than 20 mg/dl/hr)

  BS 201 to 300:   increase infusion by 1 U/hr until BS decreases to < 200

  BS 140 to 200:   do not change infusion rate

  BS 90 to 139:   decrease infusion by 1 to 2 U/hr

  BS < 90:   stop infusion; start at 1 U/hr when BS > 200

Patients with hyperosmolar nonketotic coma (HNKC) are treated with volume resuscitation. These patients usually require only small doses of insulin for glycemic control.

CHAPTER **27** _____

Renal
failure

PRERENAL AZOTEMIA (Tables 27-1 and 27-2)

Patients with prerenal azotemia (urinary Na < 40 mEq/L) should receive *aggressive fluid resuscitation*. Low-dose dopamine (2 to 5 µg/kg/min) may increase renal blood flow and reduce the risk of renal failure. Once the patient has been adequately resuscitated, a loop diuretic together with low-dose dopamine *may* attenuate the severity of the renal dysfunction.

Glomerular filtration is highly dependent on renal blood flow and renal perfusion pressure (Fig. 27-1). When both or either fall, the kidney autoregulates to maintain GFR. However, when the MAP falls below 60 mm Hg, the

Table 27-1 Laboratory data to differentiate prerenal from renal failure

Laboratory test	Prerenal	Renal
Urinalysis	Normal	Proteinuria, casts
Urinary sodium (mEq/L)	< 20	> 20
Fractional Na excretion	< 1	> 1
Urinary osmolarity	> 600	< 300
BUN/creatinine ratio	++/+	++/++

Table 27-2 Urinary findings in acute renal failure

Diagnosis	Urinary sediment
Prerenal azotemia	Normal (hyaline casts and rare granular casts)
Postrenal azotemia	Can be normal or show hematuria, pyuria, or crystals
Renal: vascular	Often has RBC; eosinophiluria can occur with atheroembolic disease
Renal: glomerulonephritis	RBC, RBC casts, and granular casts
Renal: interstitial nephritis	Pyuria, WBC casts, eosinophils, and eosinophilic casts
Renal: tubular necrosis	Pigmented granular casts, renal tubular epithelial cells, and granular casts

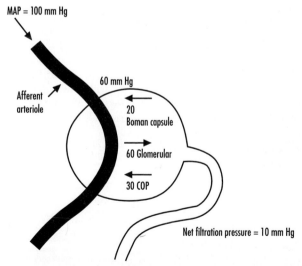

Fig. 27-1 Glomerulo filtration.

filtration pressure drops close to 0. It is therefore essential that all patients with prerenal azotemia be adequately fluid resuscitated to achieve an adequate MAP and cardiac output.

LOW-DOSE DOPAMINE: FACT OR FICTION?

Dopamine binds to DA1 and DA2 receptors in the kidney, mediating the following effects:

- Dilatation of the main renal, arcuate, and interlobar arteries and the afferent arterioles increasing renal blood flow and GFR
- Inhibits the Na-H antiport system on the brush border of the proximal convoluted tubule, causing a natriuresis
- Inhibits Na-K-ATPase on the basolateral membrane, particularly in the renal cortex, protecting the kidney from ischemia
- Direct inhibition of aldosterone

Data supporting the use of low-dose dopamine in oliguric states are conflicting. Low-dose dopamine should be limited to patients with adequate intravascular volume who, despite receiving appropriate doses of diuretics, continue to have inadequate urine output. If the patient remains oliguric, dopamine should be withdrawn.

Factors that alter the BUN/creatinine ratio

- ++BUN/+creatinine
    Dehydration
    Urinary obstruction
    Drugs—corticosteroids, tetracyclines
    Hypercatabolic conditions—sepsis
    Tissue necrosis—gangrene, burns
    Gastrointestinal bleeding
    Reduced muscle bulk
    Increased protein intake
    Urine extravasation in peritoneum

- +BUN/++creatinine
  Rhabdomyolysis
  Decreased protein intake
  Liver failure
  Increased muscle mass
  Drugs—cimetidine, cefoxitin, TMP-SMX
  Ketosis

COMMON NEPHROTOXIC AGENTS

Antibiotics

Aminoglycosides	ATN
Penicillins	Acute interstitial nephritis
Cephalosporins	Acute interstitial nephritis
Sulfamethoxazole	Acute interstitial nephritis, crystals, decreased creatinine secretion
Quinolones	?
Amphotericin B	ATN, electrolyte wasting, renal tubular acidosis
Pentamidine	ATN
Acyclovir	Crystalluria
Foscarnet	ATN, electrolyte wasting
Rifampicin	Acute interstitial nephritis

Immunosuppressive agents

Cyclosporine	Intrarenal vasoconstriction
Cisplatin	ATN
Methotrexate	Crystalluria

Antihypertensive agents

ACE inhibitors	Decreased GFR (especially with renal artery stenosis), acute interstitial nephritis

Miscellaneous

Contrast agents	ATN, acute interstitial nephritis, nephrotic syndrome
Cimetidine	Acute interstitial nephritis, decreased creatinine secretion
Allopurinol	Acute interstitial nephritis
Phenytoin	Acute interstitial nephritis
Lithium	Acute interstitial nephritis

Reducing the risk of aminoglycoside nephrotoxicity

The major limitation with the use of aminoglycoside antibiotics is nephrotoxicity. Aminoglycoside antibiotics are reported to be the most common cause of drug-induced nephrotoxicity in hospitalized patients. It is probable that between 5% and 15% of patients treated with an aminoglycoside will develop clinically significant nephrotoxicity.

- Factors that increase the risk of aminoglycoside nephrotoxicity include the following:

    More than 10 days of treatment

    A second course of aminoglycosides within 3 months of the first course

    Underlying renal dysfunction, azotemia, or renal failure. In patients with renal dysfunction, the half-life of aminoglycosides is increased, resulting in serum levels being elevated for a prolonged period. This enhances the renal uptake of the drug with increased nephrotoxicity. Furthermore, the dosage adjustments that are made in renal failure result in subtherapeutic and widely spaced peak levels in which a therapeutic failure can be predicted. Therefore, aminoglycoside antibiotics should be avoided in patients with significant renal dysfunction.

    Advanced age: increased nephrotoxicity, which has been reported in the elderly, is probably a consequence of the decreased glomerular filtration rate in this age group.

Multiple daily dosing schedule
Dehydration and prerenal azotemia
Hypokalemia and hypomagnesemia

Concurrent administration of nephrotoxic agents, especially vancomycin, amphotericin B, and cyclosporine, will increase the incidence of toxicity.

- Use the following strategy to reduce the risk of aminoglycoside toxicity:

  A once daily (qd) dosing regimen may reduce the risk of nephrotoxicity.

  In patients treated on the qd regimen, therapeutic peak levels will be achieved in almost all patients, and therefore measuring peak levels may not be needed.

  Trough levels should be measured in patients with renal dysfunction and in elderly patients (aim for a gentamicin/tobramycin trough < 1.0 and preferably < 0.5 µg/ml)

  Limit duration of "course" to 7 to 10 days

  Avoid using in patients with underlying renal disease

Reducing the risk of contrast-induced renal toxicity

- Diabetics, dehydrated patients, and patients with underlying renal disease are at an increased risk of developing contrast-induced renal failure.
- Patients receiving intravenous contrast agents should be prehydrated before the procedure to ensure a good urine output. The value of using mannitol and furosemide together with fluid loading is unproven.

RHABDOMYLOSIS AND MYOGLOBINURIA

Rhabdomyolysis with myoglobinuria is commonly encountered in the ICU. Causes include the following:

- Crush injury
- Compartment syndrome

- Ischemic limb
- Severe sepsis
- Cocaine use
- Hypothermia
- Unconscious patients lying in one position
- Alcohol

Damage to skeletal muscle cells results in the bidirectional flow of solutes and water across the cell membrane with hypovolemia, hypocalcemia, hyperkalemia, hyperphosphatemia, and a metabolic acidosis.

- Influx from extracellular compartment
    Water and NaCl
    Calcium
- Efflux from damaged muscle cells
    Potassium
    Purines
    Phosphate
    Lactic and other organic acids
    Myoglobin
    Thromboplastin
    Creatinine phosphokinase
    Creatinine

Rhabdomyolysis should be suspected in a patient with high levels of CPK MM and confirmed by demonstrating myoglobin in the urine. Patients with a CPK greater than 10,000 U/ml are at a high risk of developing acute renal failure. The CPKs should be serially followed since levels may rise with volume resuscitation (and increased muscle perfusion). All dehydrated patients with elevated CPKs should be rehydrated. Patients with CPKs above 5000 should be aggressively treated to prevent renal failure.

- Maintain a urine output of 100 to 200 ml/hr with fluid replacement (NaCl or Ringer's) and the use of a loop diuretic.
- Alkalinize the urine (IV sodium bicarbonate).
- Mannitol may also be useful to maintain a high urine output (check osmolarity regularly).

- Monitor fluid balance carefully; do not dehydrate or overload the patient.
- Hypocalcemia is a common complication of rhabdomyolysis. Release of phosphate from injured muscle results in the local precipitation of calcium salts. Hyperphosphatemia also impairs the 1-hydroxylation of vitamin D, thereby decreasing the sensitivity of bone to parathormone. Administration of calcium may result in severe soft tissue calcification. Calcium supplementation should be reserved for patients with clear clinical signs of hypocalcemia. In patients receiving hemodialysis the dialysate calcium should be adjusted to prevent a positive calcium balance.

MANAGEMENT OF AZOTEMIA, OLIGURIA, AND ESTABLISHED ACUTE RENAL FAILURE

$$\text{Est CrCl} = [(140 - \text{age}) \times \text{wt(kg)} / \text{plasma creatinine} \times 70] \{\text{women} \times 0.85\}$$

Rule 1: always catheterize the patient to exclude a full bladder

Rule 2: a renal ultrasound should be performed in all patients with ARF to exclude obstruction

Rule 3: always check the urine for casts, eosinophils, etc.

Once the patient is in established acute renal failure, loop diuretics and dopamine are of little value. Nephrotoxic agents such as aminoglycoside antibiotics and contrast agents should be avoided at all costs.

There are no hard and fast rules about when renal replacement therapy (dialysis) should be instituted. However, in the critically ill patient with rapid changes in fluid balance and electrolytes, it is usually prudent to start sooner rather than later. Except in unusual circumstances, continuous renal replacement therapy (i.e., continuous arteriovenous hemofiltration [CAVH], continuous arteriovenous hemodialysis [CAVHD], continuous venoveno hemodialysis [CVVHD]) with slow, continuous ultrafiltration (SCUF) is the treatment of choice. This method of renal replacement therapy is the most physiologic and is the best method for regulating fluid and electrolyte balance in the critically ill ICU patient.

The standard criteria for initiating renal replacement therapy include the following:

- Hyperkalemia (K > 6.5 mmol/L)
- Progressive acidosis with pH < 7.25
- Fluid overload with pulmonary edema
- Pericardial effusion
- Uremic symptoms, i.e., nausea, vomiting, altered mental status, asterixis
- Increase of serum creatinine > 2 mg/dl/day

CONTINUOUS RENAL REPLACEMENT THERAPY IN ACUTE RENAL FAILURE

Advantages of continuous renal replacement therapy include the following:

- Hemodynamically well tolerated
- Minimal change in plasma osmolarity
- Better control of azotemia and electrolytes and acid-base balance
- Very effective in removing fluid
- Technically simple
- Membrane capable of removing cytokines in septic patients
- Better membrane biocompatibility

Continuous renal replacement therapies have been developed to enable the critically ill patient with acute renal failure to be treated more effectively. Acute renal failure in the critically ill patient almost always develops in the setting of shock, sepsis, major surgery, and/or major trauma, and it is invariably associated with multiorgan dysfunction or failure. In addition, these patients usually have hemodynamic and respiratory abnormalities that make conventional intermittent hemodialysis both technically difficult and fraught with many complications. The patient's fluid, electrolyte, and acid-base status fluctuate widely within a 24-hour period; intermittent dialysis is not suited to these changing circumstances.

Continuous renal replacement therapies were developed with the aim of providing a more physiologic method of renal replacement therapy, i.e., to function more like a normal kidney. A number of methods have been described; however, they are largely variations of the same theme.

Continuous arteriovenous hemofiltration (CAVH) was the first continuous renal replacement therapy to be used in ICU patients. Essentially, this is a method of continuously removing a plasma ultrafiltrate and replacing the lost volume with a balanced physiologic solution. A hollow fiber filter (the artificial kidney) is connected at one end to an arterial catheter (usually the femoral artery) and to a venous catheter at the other end (usually the femoral vein), forming a closed-loop system. The patient's own cardiac output perfuses the filter (there are no external pumps). Heparin is added to the arterial end to prevent clotting of blood in the filter. The blood flow through the system is dependent on the cardiac output, mean arterial pressure, and the diameter and length of the connecting tubes.

The CAVH and CAVHD filters have a larger surface area, larger pore size, and higher hydraulic permeability than do the conventional cellulose hemodialysis filters, enhancing the ultrafiltration process. In addition, the membranes have improved biocompatibility and do not activate the complement system. Hydrostatic pressure forces plasma water out of the blood compartment in the extravascular filtrate compartment. The filtrate flows through a collecting tube to a closed drainage compartment below the level of the patient. This negative pressure adds to the positive pressure exerted across the filter membrane, enhancing the filtration process. The rate of ultrafiltration is therefore dependent on the blood flow through the kidney, the mean arterial pressure, and the distance the collecting container is below the level of the patient. A mean arterial pressure above 60 mm Hg is required to maintain flow through the system.

The concentrations of most solutes in the filtrate are approximately the same as those in the plasma. Hence this is a method of ultrafiltration and not dialysis. The filtration rate is approximately 10 ml/min or 600 ml/hr. This method is therefore very efficient in removing fluid but insufficient to control azotemia in hypercatabolic patients with acute renal failure.

To improve the solute clearance and better control azotemia while retaining the advances of slow, continuous therapy, a more efficient diffusion-based therapy known as *CAVHD* (continuous arteriovenous hemodialysis) was developed. This method is currently the *therapy of choice* for acute renal failure in the critically ill patient. This system allows for diffusion (dialysis) and convection (ultrafiltration) to occur simultaneously. The extracorporeal circuitry is basically similar to that in CAVH, except that dialysate is infused through the dialysate compartment (Fig. 27-2). A dual-chamber peristaltic infusion pump allows one to propel dialysate through one end of the dialysate compartment and pump dialysate and ultrafiltrate out through the other end. The dialysate inflow rate is usually set at about 1000 ml/hr. Using this system, one can "electronically" determine the hourly net "urine" output (difference between the rate of the two pumps).

The dialysate flow is about 15 ml/min (3% of the value with conventional hemodialysis), while the blood flow is approximately 100 ml/min. This results in the presentation of a large quantity of blood solute to the highly permeable membrane. As a consequence, the concentration of small blood solutes exiting the dialyzer is approximately equal to the solute concentration of the plasma entering the dialyzer. The clearance of CAVHD is approximately 21 ml/min.

Because the CAVHD filter is a foreign membrane, heparin is required to prevent clotting of the filter. Clotting of the kidney is the single biggest problem with this continuous extracorporeal system. Because of the relatively slow flow rate, the filter will clot if the blood is not adequately anticoagulated. However, the use of heparin can be prob-

lematic in ICU patients who often have a preexistent coagulopathy. Therefore careful attention to the adequacy of
anticoagulation is required to prolong the life of the filter
and at the same time reduce the risk of bleeding. A bedside, automated, activated clotting-time apparatus (e.g.,
Hemacron) is strongly recommended. Heparin is usually
started at 500 IU/hr and titrated to achieve an arterial
PTT between 40 and 50 seconds and a Hemacron clotting
time of between 150 and 200 seconds.

The dosages of drugs must be adjusted according to
the estimated clearance. In addition, as amino acids are fil-
tered out by the filter, the amount of amino acid content
of TPN solutions should be increased by approximately
20% (Tables 27-3 and 27-4).

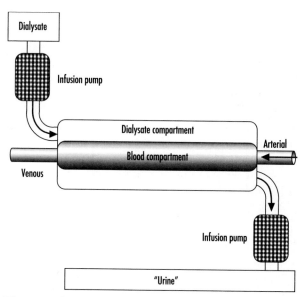

Fig. 27-2 Schematic drawing of continuous arteriovenous
hemodialysis (CAVHD).

Table 27-3 Urea clearance with various renal replacement modalities

Urea clearance	CAVHD	CAVH	Peritoneal dialysis	Standard dialysis	Intermittent dialysis for 3.5 hr, 5 day/week
K urea (ml/min)	21	10	17	15	22

Table 27-4 Common drugs used in the ICU that require dosage adjustment in renal failure

Drug	Dose based on estimated CrCl		
	> 50	10-50	< 10
Opiates	Unchanged	Unchanged	50% to 75%
Chlordiazepoxide	Unchanged	Unchanged	50%
Lorazepam	Unchanged	Unchanged	50%
Ceftazidime	Unchanged	50	25%
Ceftizoxime	Unchanged	50	25%

Cefuroxime	Unchanged	50	25%
Other cephalosporins	Unchanged	Unchanged	50%
Most penicillins	Unchanged	50-75	25%
Ciprofloxacin	Unchanged	50	25%
Erythromycin	Unchanged	Unchanged	50% to 75%
Tri/Sulp	Unchanged	75	50%
Vancomycin	Monitor levels		
Aminoglycosides	75-50 monitor levels	*Avoid*	*Avoid*
Carbamazepine	Unchanged	Unchanged	75%
Amphotericin B	Unchanged	Unchanged	75%
Fluconazole	Unchanged	50	25%
Acyclovir	Unchanged	50	25%
H$_2$-blockers	Unchanged	75	50%
Atenolol	Unchanged	50	25%
Allopurinol	Unchanged	50	25%
Chlorpropamide	Unchanged	*Avoid*	*Avoid*

CHAPTER 28

Thyroid disease

TOXIC CRISIS (THYROID STORM)

Diagnosis

- Exaggerated signs and symptoms of thyrotoxicosis
- Rectal temperature > 101° F
- Tachycardia > 100 beats/min

Treatment

- *Supportive measures*: fluid and electrolyte resuscitation
- *Treatment of hyperthermia*: acetaminophen, alcohol sponges, cooling blankets
- IV beta-blockade titrated to pulse; propranolol 1 to 2 mg IV boluses, metoprolol 5 mg boluses or esmolol titration
- Stress doses of corticosteroids
- Propylthiouracil 200 to 250 mg PO q 4 hr
- Iodine, started 1 hour after first dose of propylthiouracil

  Sodium ipodate (iodine-containing contrast agent used for gallbladder imaging), 1 to 3 g PO q day, 1 to 3 days

  Lugol's iodine 30 drops/day

MYXEDEMA CRISIS

Diagnosis

The diagnosis of myxedema is made on clinical grounds

(exaggerated features of hypothyroidism) supported by thyroid function tests.

Treatment

- Treat the precipitating cause(s), i.e., sepsis, dehydration, electrolyte disturbances, etc.
- *Supportive measures*: hypothermia should not be treated with warming blankets (can precipitate cardiovascular collapse)
- Thyroxine 300 to 500 μg IV followed by 100 μg/day until the patient can take orally
- Stress doses of corticosteroids (hydrocortisone 100 mg q 8 hr)

SICK EUTHYROID SYNDROME

Alterations in thyroid physiology that occur in the critically ill patient are referred to as the *sick euthyroid syndrome*. The interpretation of thyroid function tests in these patients is extremely complex. Hyperthyroidism, however, is not difficult to diagnose clinically or by thyroid function testing. The important question, however, is which patients are hypothyroidic and require treatment and which patients are euthyroidic? As can be seen from Table 28-1, this distinction can be very difficult to make.

Table 28-1 Profile of thyroid hormones during acute illness

Phase of illness	T3	T4	FT4	rT3	TSH
Mild, early	D	N	N	I	N
Moderate	D	N,D	N	I	N
Severe	D	D	D	I	N,D
Early recovery	D	D,N	D,N	I	N,I

D, Decreased; *I*, increased; *N*, normal.

Generally, unless there are obvious signs and symptoms of hypothyroidism, the patient should not receive thyroid replacement therapy. Thyroid function tests, however, should be repeated once the patient recovers from the acute illness.

CHAPTER 29

Corticosteroids and adrenal insufficiency

Refer to Table 29-1.

DELETERIOUS EFFECTS OF CORTICOSTEROID THERAPY

- Immunologic

  Suppresses immune surveillance

  Effects neutrophil and lymphocyte proliferation and function

  Affects cytokine production, e.g., decreases TNF, IL-1, and IL-2 production

  Affects production of local mediators, such as prostaglandins and leukotrienes

  Decreases antibody production
- Hematologic

  Neutrophilia

  Erythrocytosis and thrombocytosis

  Lymphopenia

  Monocytopenia
- Metabolic

  Hyperglycemia (hepatic gluconeogenesis and inhibition of peripheral glucose utilization)

  Peripheral protein catabolism

  Altered lipid metabolism

Table 29-1 Properties of commonly used corticosteroids

Agent	Equivalent dose (mg)	Glucocorticoid potency	Mineralocorticoid potency	Duration of action (hr)
Dexamethasone	0.75	25	0	72
Methylprednisolone	4	5	0.5	36
Prednisolone	5	4	0.8	24
Prednisone	5	4	0.8	24
Hydrocortisone	25	1	1	8

Poor wound healing

Suppression of the hypothalamic-pituitary-adrenal axis

Hypokalemic metabolic alkalosis
- Cardiovascular

Cardiovascular collapse and sudden death with rapid IV administration

Hypertension

Sodium and fluid retention
- Musculoskeletal

Proximal myopathy

Osteoporosis

Aseptic necrosis of bones, especially femoral head

Respiratory muscle myopathy

Associated with prolonged neuromuscular failure in patients who concomitantly received prolonged neuromuscular blocking agents
- Gastrointestinal

Delayed healing of peptic ulceration, with an increased risk of bleeding and perforation

Pancreatitis
- Central nervous system

Euphoria

Psychosis
- Ophthalmologic

Ocular hypertension

Subcapsular cataracts
- Dermatologic

Hirsutism

Atrophy of skin and subcutaneous tissue

INDICATIONS FOR CORTICOSTEROID THERAPY IN THE ICU

As can be seen from the list above, corticosteroid therapy is associated with severe and sometimes life-threatening complications. Corticosteroids are among the most abused group of drugs used in the ICU. Corticosteroids should only be used when absolutely indicated, and then in an appropriate dosage schedule.

- *Proven* indications for steroids include the following:
  Asthma
  Acute exacerbation of COPD
  Chronic COPD patients who demonstrate an improvement in symptoms and/or pulmonary function tests after a trial of steroids

  Anaphylactic and acute allergic reactions
  Active vasculitic disease, collagen vascular diseases
  Allergic bronchopulmonary aspergillosis
  Bronchiolitis obliterans organizing pneumonia (BOOP)

  Superior vena caval syndrome caused by malignancy
  Acute spinal cord injury
  Acute bacterial meningitis in *pediatric patients*
  Autoimmune hemolytic anemia
  ITP in adults
  Tuberculous meningitis and pericarditis, and possibly tuberculous pleural effusions

  HIV-positive patients with *Pneumocystis carinii* with PaO_2 on room air < 70 mm Hg

  Adrenal insufficiency, Addison syndrome, and Waterhouse-Friderichsen syndrome

  Chronic phase of ARDS (fibroproliferative phase)
  Pemphigus, pemphigoid, erythema multiforme, toxic epidermolysis

  Severe acute alcoholic hepatitis
  In oncologic patients, as part of the chemotherapeutic regimen or antinausea regimen

  In hypercalcemia caused by carcinoma of breast and myeloma

Crohn disease and ulcerative colitis
In the treatment of patients with cerebral tumors
Hypereosinophilia syndromes
Together with praziquantel in cerebral cysticercosis
- Conditions for which steroids have been *proven to be of no value*
Sepsis syndrome and septic shock
Acute phase of ARDS
Prophylaxis of ARDS
Malaria
Head injury
Raised intracranial pressure, *except* as a result of tumor masses, cerebral cystercicosis

Acute myocardial infarction
Acute bacterial pneumonia

ADRENAL INSUFFICIENCY

- Patients who have been on oral corticosteroids, equivalent to 5 mg methylprednisolone for longer than 10 days, will have suppression of the hypothalamic-pituitary-adrenal axis and will require steroid supplementation during stress
- Patients with Addison disease will require steroid supplementation
- Patients with relative adrenal insufficiency may be unmasked during an acute illness and may require steroid supplementation. A high index of suspicion should exist in the following situations:
Shock refractory to fluid and inotropic resuscitation
Patients with malignancy
HIV-positive patients
Patients with other autoimmune diseases, including diabetes

Septicemia
Malnourished patients

- Patients may develop acute adrenal insufficiency because of adrenal hemorrhage or necrosis, e.g., in septicemic patients, especially meningococcemia.
- In acute or subacute adrenal insufficiency, patients rarely present with the classic features of hyperkalemia and hyponatremia.
- The normal *physiologic* replacement dose of corticosteroid is equal to 30 mg hydrocortisone daily (20 mg in the morning and 10 mg in the evening).
- During maximal stress, the daily corticosteroid production is equal to approximately 300 mg hydrocortisone.
- *If there is a high index of suspicion, patients should be treated with dexamethasone (4 mg q 8 hr), until the ACTH stimulation test has been performed.*

Diagnosis of adrenal insufficiency

In a critically ill patient a random plasma cortisol level of less than 10 µg/ml is almost diagnostic of adrenal insufficiency.

An ACTH stimulation test is easy to perform and should probably be done in all patients with suspected adrenal insufficiency.

A baseline serum cortisol is drawn

250 µg of synthetic ACTH (Cortrosyn) is injected

A 1-hour serum cortisol level is drawn

Normally a rise of serum cortisol of at least 7 µg/dl should occur, and the level should rise to > 18 µg/dl by 60 minutes (Fig. 29-1).

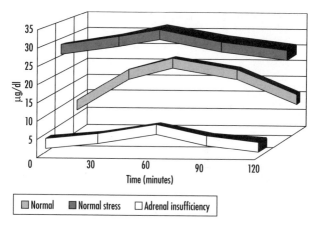

Fig. 29-1 ACTH stimulation test.

PART FOUR

THE GASTROINTESTINAL TRACT

CHAPTER 30

Liver failure and dysfunction

CAUSES OF JAUNDICE IN THE ICU PATIENT

- Prehepatic (> 15% conjugated bilirubin)
  Blood transfusions
  Blood resorption from hematomas
  G6PD deficiency
  Sickle cell disease
  Hemolysis secondary to sepsis
- "Noncholestatic" hepatocellular dysfunction
  "Shock liver" from prolonged hypotension, especially if underlying cardiac failure exists

  Postcardiopulmonary bypass
  Drugs
    Direct hepatotoxicity
    Hypersensitive reactions
  Hepatitis
    Viral
    Alcoholic
- Cholestatic and hepatocellular dysfunction
  Benign postoperative cholestasis
  TPN
  Sepsis/MSOF
- Obstructive (> 40% conjugated bilirubin)
  Acalculous cholecystitis
  Choledocholithiasis
  Pancreatitis

CAUSES OF FULMINANT HEPATIC FAILURE

- Viral hepatitis
  Hepatitis B, C, and E, and rarely A and D infection
  CMV infection
  Viral hemorrhagic fevers
- Drugs and toxins
  Acetaminophen
  Alcohol
  Isoniazid
  Valproic acid
  Phenytoin
  Amanita phalloides
  Carbon tetrachloride
- Miscellaneous
  Fatty liver of pregnancy
  Reye syndrome
  Wilson disease
  Autoimmune chronic active hepatitis
  Budd-Chiari syndrome (especially in patients with underlying hepatic disease)

STAGES OF HEPATIC ENCEPHALOPATHY

Stage 1: mild confusion, slowed mentation, slurred speech, mild asterixis

Stage 2: drowsiness, inappropriate behavior, marked asterixis

Stage 3: marked confusion; patient sleeps most of the time but is rousable; asterixis present

Stage 4: deep coma

MANAGEMENT OF HEPATIC FAILURE

- Elevate head of bed 20 to 35 degrees
- Monitor blood glucose; 5% to 10% DW to prevent hypoglycemia
- Monitor volume status, urine output

- Exclude or treat sepsis
- Exclude or treat upper GI bleeding
- *Avoid* sedative and hypnotic drugs (benzodiazepines are notorious for precipitating hepatic encephalopathy)
- Lactulose titrated to produce 2 to 4 loose stools per day
- Vitamin 10 mg IV first 3 days
- High-protein, high-calorie enteral feeding (see Chapter 52)
- FFP/fibrinogen for active bleeding
- Corticosteroids are indicated in patients with severe alcoholic hepatitis
- Mannitol 0.5 mg/kg in patients in stage 4 encephalopathy (who do not have renal failure or azotemia). Monitor volume status, electrolytes, and osmolarity very carefully. Keep osmol < 320 mosml/L
- Raised ICP is present in most patients with fulminant liver failure and is the commonest cause of death. Therapeutic interventions based on ICP monitoring have not been shown to change the outcome of FHF. However, ICP monitoring may be useful in patients who are being considered for liver transplant

CHAPTER 31

Pancreatitis

RANSON CRITERIA FOR GRADING THE SEVERITY OF PANCREATITIS

- On admission, assess the following:
    Age > 55
    Blood glucose > 200 mg/dl
    WBC > 16×10^9/L
    SGOT > 120 IU/L
    LDH > 350 IU/L
- During the first 48 hours:
    Fall in HCT > 10%
    Serum calcium < 8.0 mEq/L
    Base deficit > 4 mEq/L
    Blood urea increase > 5 mg/dl
    Fluid sequestration > 6 L
    Arterial Po_2 < 60 mm Hg

TREATMENT

- Fluid resuscitation and correction of electrolytes imbalances
- *Therapy for pain*: meperidine IM or IV or fentanyl
- NPO
- Monitor intravascular volume, clinical and PCWP

- Monitor arterial blood gases and/or pulse oximetry
- Nasogastric suction only in patients with an ileus or vomiting
- Broad-spectrum antibiotics with anaerobic cover in severe pancreatitis, e.g., imipenem (reduces risk of pancreatic abscess)
- TPN, when prolonged NPO anticipated (see Chapter 52)
    IV lipids are safe if TG is monitored
      TG < 400 mg/dl during infusion
      TG < 200 mg/dl after infusion
    Preliminary data suggest that duodenal/jejunal feeding with a low-fat elemental diet does not stimulate pancreatic secretions and may be safe in pancreatitis
- Therapeutic peritoneal lavage is of no value
- Necrosectomy and lavage if pancreas necrotic or abscess develops
- *Somatostatin*: acute pancreatitis is caused by the activation of pancreatic enzymes that autodigest the pancreas. Inhibition of pancreatic secretions is therefore a possible treatment modality. The use of somatostatin and its analogues in the treatment of acute pancreatitis is somewhat controversial. However, a metaanalysis of a number of trials has shown that somatostatin reduces the complication rate and the mortality (see Chapter 32)

COMPLICATIONS

- Abdominal
    Pancreatic necrosis
    Pancreatic abscess
    Pseudocyst
    Intraperitoneal hemorrhage
    Splenic vein thrombosis
    Obstructive jaundice

- Systemic

    Pulmonary—ARDS, pleural effusion, atelectasis, pneumonia

    DIC/coagulopathy
    Upper GI bleeding
    Acute renal failure
    Metabolic—hypocalcemia, hyperglycemia, hypertriglyceridemia

Upper GI bleeding

INITIAL ASSESSMENT AND MANAGEMENT OF UPPER GI BLEEDING

- The urgency with which GI bleeding is managed is dictated by the rate of bleeding.

  The patient with trace heme-positive stools and without severe anemia can be managed as an outpatient.

  Visible blood requires hospitalization and inpatient evaluation.

  Persistent bleeding or rebleed with hemodynamic instability necessitates ICU admission.

  Massive bleeding is defined as a loss of 30% or more of estimated blood volume or bleeding requiring blood transfusion of 6 or more units in a 24-hour period.
- *Hemodynamic assessment*: blood pressure, pulse, postural changes and assessment of peripheral perfusion.
- *Estimating blood loss*: this can be estimated by measuring the return from a NG tube. An approximate estimate of blood loss can be made by the hemodynamic response to a 2 L crystalloid fluid challenge.

  If BP returns to normal and stabilizes, blood loss of 15% to 30% has occurred.

If BP rises but falls again, blood volume loss of 30% to 40% has occurred.

If BP continues to fall, blood volume loss of > 40% has probably occurred.

- Resuscitation

  Establish two large-bore IV lines or a large-bore central line

  Insert NG tube and aspiration (by hand)
  Volume expansion with colloid and crystalloid

  Cross match blood: transfuse if large blood loss or patient is hemodynamically unstable. Give FFP after 6 units of PRBCs and platelets after 10 units

  Monitor BP, pulse, and urine output
- *History and examination*: attempt to localize the most likely source of bleeding.
- All patients with upper GI bleeding should have endoscopy performed once the patient has been adequately resuscitated. Endoscopy allows a diagnosis to be made, the risk of rebleeding to be determined, and allows for a therapeutic procedure to be performed, (i.e., sclerotherapy, banding, electrocoagulation).

MANAGEMENT OF BLEEDING PEPTIC ULCERS

- No evidence that gastric lavage will stop bleeding or prevent rebleeding
- No evidence that vasoconstrictors, such as vasopressin or somatostatin, are of any benefit
- No evidence that agents that reduce gastric acidity have any impact on actively bleeding ulcers or on the risk of rebleeding. However, most patients are treated with a continuous infusion of an H_2-blocker (cimetidine 900 mg infusion over 24 hours).
- Bipolar electrocoagulation and heat probe therapy are two promising endoscopic techniques for achieving endoscopic hemostasis

MANAGEMENT OF ESOPHAGEAL VARICES

- *Volume resuscitation*: use colloids because excess crystalloids will exacerbate ascites; avoid overhydration
- Correction of clotting factors
- *NG intubation*: evacuate blood and monitor bleeding
- *Somatostatin*: infusion 250 μg/hr (more effective than vasopressin) *or*
- *Vasopressin*: loading dose of 20 U over 20 minutes followed by 0.4 U/min and nitroglycerin at 40 μg/min; monitor for cardiac and limb ischemia
- *Sclerotherapy*: will control bleeding in 85% to 90% of patients
- *Balloon tamponade in uncontrolled bleeding (Sengstaken-Blakemore tube)*: this is a temporizing measure to control bleeding. It is associated with significant morbidity and should only be used in patients with ongoing, uncontrolled bleeding
- Decompressive shunts (Table 32-1)
    TIPS: transjugular intrahepatic portosystemic shunt—percutaneous method of achieving a side-to-side shunt

    Side-to-side portal systemic shunt
    Selective variceal decompression

BIOLOGIC EFFECTS OF SOMATOSTATIN

- *Endocrine effects* inhibit secretion of the following:
    Gastrin
    Pancreozymin
    Secretin
    Human pancreatic peptide
    Vasoactive intestinal peptide
    Gastric inhibitory peptide
    Motilin
    Glucagon
    Insulin
    Cholecystokinin

Lipase
Amylase
Trypsin
Growth hormone
TSH
- *Nonendocrine effects* inhibit the following:
    Gastric acid secretion and emptying
    Pancreatic secretion
    Gallbladder contraction
    Splanchnic blood flow
    Intestinal transit
    Macronutrient absorption

Table 32-1 Child's criteria (surgical risk for shunting)

Variable	Group A	Group B	Group C
S-bilirubin (mg/dl)	< 2	2-3	> 3
S-albumin (g%)	> 3.5	3.0-3.5	< 3.0
Ascites	None	Easily controlled	Poorly controlled
Neurologic disorder	None	Minimal	Comatose
Nutrition	Excellent	Good	Poor

CHAPTER 33

GI prophylaxis

GI PROPHYLAXIS

Refer to Fig. 33-1.

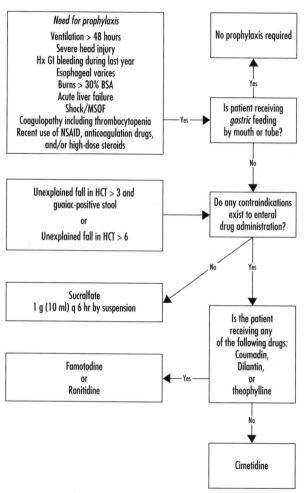

Fig. 33-1 Gastrointestinal (GI) prophylaxis.

PART FIVE

NEUROLOGY

Seizures

TREATMENT OF STATUS EPILEPTICUS

Refer to Fig. 34-1 and Table 34-1.

Phenytoin

Phenytoin is the most commonly used anticonvulsant in the ICU, and therefore an understanding of the pharmacokinetics and pharmacodynamics of this drug is important.

- Phenytoin is metabolized by the liver and follows zero-order kinetics, i.e., the metabolic process is saturable, and therefore doubling the dose *does not* double the serum concentration (the serum concentration increases exponentially). A small increase in the

Table 34-1 Anticonvulsant drugs

Drug	Serum level (µg/ml)	Daily dose (mg)
Phenytoin	10-20 total 1-2 free fraction	4 mg/kg/day 200-500
Carbamazepine	4-12	600-2400
Phenobarbital	15-45	60-300
Ethosuximide	40-100	500-1500
Valproic acid	50-100	750-3000

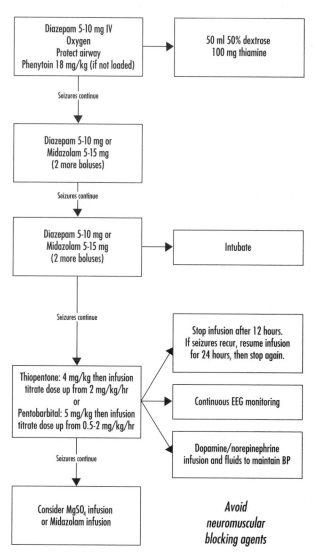

Fig. 34-1 Generalized seizures.

dose may result in a large increase in serum levels (into the toxic range).

- Phenytoin is 90% protein bound. Only the free fraction is pharmacologically active. Critically ill patients frequently have a decreased serum albumin concentration, which increases the free phenytoin fraction (may cause toxicity). The therapeutic concentration (10 to 20 µg/ml) reflects both the bound and unbound fractions. Therefore in hypoalbuminemic patients, the free phenytoin concentration should be monitored (1 to 2 µg/ml).

- Drugs that cause autoinduction of hepatic enzymes increase phenytoin clearance, whereas drugs that inhibit hepatic enzymes cause phenytoin clearance to decline.

    Drugs that increase phenytoin metabolism include the following:
        Barbiturates
        Ethanol
        Folic acid
        Rifampin
        Trimethoprim
    Drugs that decrease phenytoin metabolism include the following:
        Chloramphenicol
        Disulfiram
        Isoniazid
        Phenylbutazone

- IV loading dose
    18 to 20 mg/kg, lean body weight
    No faster than 50 mg/min
    Give only in 0.9 NaCl (insoluble in D_5W)
    May cause hypotension, bradycardia, heart block, arrhythmias, and asystole (particularly if infused too rapidly)

    Contraindicated in patients with second- or third-degree heart block

An external pacemaker should be available in patients with conduction abnormalities

- Toxicity

    Ataxia, nausea, vomiting, nystagmus, involuntary movements, confusion, hallucinations

    Hypersensitivity reactions, including skin rashes, hepatitis, fever, Stevens-Johnson syndrome, and the dilantin hypersensitivity syndrome

CHAPTER 35

Subarachnoid hemorrhage

HUNT AND HESS CLASSIFICATION

Grade	Characteristics
I	Asymptomatic or slight headache
II	Moderate to severe headache, nuchal rigidity, no neurologic deficit other than cranial nerve palsy
III	Drowsiness, confusion, or mild focal deficit
IV	Stupor, moderate to severe hemiparesis
V	Deep coma, decerebrate rigidity

MANAGEMENT (see also Chapter 37)

- Head elevation of 20 to 35 degrees
- Hypertension should be treated very cautiously and keep systolic pressure between 120 and 150 mm Hg; labetalol is probably drug of choice.
- Anxiolysis or sedation for grades I and II
- *Pain management*: morphine sulphate, codeine, or meperidine
- Maintain euvolemia; dehydration reduces preload, cardiac output, and cerebral perfusion thereby increasing risk of cerebral infarction
- Laxative
- DVT prophylaxis (stockings or pneumatic boots)

- Mannitol 0.25 g/kg q 4 to 6 hours if ICP is raised (clinical assessment or directly measured). Osmolarity should not exceed 320 mosm/L
- Ventriculostomy for acute hydrocephalus
- Prevention of cerebral vasospasm; nimodipine 60 mg q 4 to 6 hours
- *Surgical management*: grades I to III should undergo surgery as soon as possible

VASOPLASM COMPLICATING SUBARACHNOID HEMORRHAGE

- Diagnosed by change in mental status 3 to 10 days after bleeding not caused by another neurologic complication and confirmed by angiography or transcranial Doppler
- Hypervolemic hemodilution or induced arterial hypertension has been shown to be of benefit in uncontrolled reports
- Angioplasty of the implicated vessel has also been reported

CHAPTER 36

Cerebrovascular disease

MANAGEMENT

- There are no data to suggest that admitting patients with an acute cerebrovascular accident to an intensive care unit improves outcome.
- Patients require good nursing care in a "stroke unit."
- In the hypertensive patient, the blood pressure should not be treated in the early stages of the cerebrovascular accident unless the systolic is > 220 mm Hg or the diastolic > 120 mm Hg, and then very cautiously.
- Surgical decompression may be indicated in patients with large posterior fossa bleeds or infarcts.
- Ventriculostomy may be indicated in patients with an obstructive hydrocephalus from an intraventricular bleed.
- Corticosteroids are of no benefit; they only increase the complication rate.
- Calcium channel blockers are of marginal benefit; NMDA (N-methyl-D-aspartate) receptor blockers may prove to be more beneficial.
- Mannitol and hyperventilation may be used in patients with evidence of raised ICP on CT; there is, however, very little data to show that this intervention improves outcome.
- Patients with atrial fibrillation who are suspected to have suffered an embolic stroke should undergo a

repeat CT scan at about 72 hours. If the infarct is nonhemorrhagic, anticoagulation with heparin should be instituted.

- Patients with no gag reflex should be fed with a feeding tube or a jejunostomy tube.

CHAPTER 37

Closed head injury

GLASGOW COMA SCALE

The Glasgow Coma Scale should be recorded for all patients since it has important prognostic and therapeutic significance.

Sign	Finding	Value
Eye opening	Spontaneous	4
	To voice	3
	To pain	2
	None	1
Verbal response	Orientated	5
	Confused	4
	Inappropriate	3
	Incomprehensible	2
	None	1
Motor response	Obeys commands	6
	Localizes to pain	5
	Withdraws from pain	4
	Flexion	3
	Extension	2
	None	1

MANAGEMENT

General measures

- The injured brain is extremely vulnerable to both systemic and local insults. For this reason, a pro-active approach to head injury is essential.
- The patient's level of consciousness and presence of focal neurologic signs should be documented.
- The patient must be thoroughly examined to exclude the possibility of other injuries.
- Endotracheal intubation is recommended to maintain the airway and facilitate ventilation in all patients with a decreased level of consciousness.
- A CT scan (plus x-ray of cervical spine) is essential for all patients who have a history of loss of consciousness or who have a depressed level of consciousness, skull fracture, and/or focal neurologic signs.
- Sedate (cautiously) if patient is restless.
- Early enteral nutrition
- DVT prophylaxis
- Corticosteroids are *contraindicated.* Five randomized, prospective clinical trials have convincingly demonstrated that high-dose glucocorticoid therapy is ineffective in altering the course of intracranial hypertension or improving neurologic outcome. Glucocorticoids, however, increase the complication rate in these patients. In addition, animal data suggest that steroids may be "toxic" to damaged neurons.
- Prophylactic anticonvulsant therapy (phenytoin) has been demonstrated to reduce the risk of posttraumatic seizures during the first week after injury. Prophylactic treatment with anticonvulsants for more than 7 days is controversial.
- Fever should be actively treated in the head-injured patient with acetaminophen and a cooling blanket if necessary (the source should be identified and treated).

Management of intracranial hematomas

- Urgent evacuation is required in all extracerebral hematomas that are associated with 5 mm or more midline shift and/or are more than 25 ml or more in calculated volume.
- In patients with "small" extracerebral hematomas, it is essential to repeat the CT after a few hours in all patients in whom the first CT was carried out within 6 hours of injury.

Management of raised intracranial pressure (ICP)

- Significant increase in ICP occurs in over 50% of patients with severe head injury during the first 72 hours.
- *ICP monitoring*: although not proven to change the outcome, ICP monitoring is currently recommended for patients with a GCS of between 5 and 9. *It can also be used to guide therapy and to minimize the multiple risks adherent to the treatment modalities of intracranial hypertension.* ICP monitoring may also be indicated in the following circumstances:

  Obliteration of the third ventricle and basal cisterns on CT

  Patients with subdural or epidural hematomas
  Patients with midline shift

- Continuous monitoring of jugular venous saturation may provide useful information in patients with severe head injuries.
- *The cerebral perfusion pressure (MAP-ICP) should be kept at 70 mm Hg or higher.* The ICP should ideally be kept below 20 mm Hg. *Some investigators have suggested that keeping the ICP below 15 mm Hg may improve outcome.* Moderate increases to 25 mm Hg or even 30 mm Hg may be tolerated, provided the cerebral perfusion pressure is above 70 mm Hg.

  CSF drainage, mannitol, and pressors should be used in conjunction to treat both the intracranial pressure and the systemic arterial side of the components of the CPP equation.

Mannitol 0.25 g/kg q 4 to 8 hours (*should be given as intermittent boluses and not as a constant infusion*). Check osmolarity q 8 to 12 hours and maintain less than 310 mosm/L (*there is no benefit in increasing the serum osmol above 310 mosm/L*).

The patient should be kept euvolemic. There are no data demonstrating that dehydration reduces brain water. Dehydration may, however, reduce preload, cardiac output, and cerebral perfusion.

Vasopressors may be required to maintain an adequate MAP. These agents are almost always required in patients in a barbiturate coma. Norepinephrine and/or dopamine may be used in this circumstance.

Ventilate the patient to maintain the Pa_{CO_2} at *33 to 37* mm Hg; although hyperventilation is initially effective for ICP control, its efficiency remains limited to short periods (less than 4 hours). Severe alkalosis may decrease cerebral flow and induce cerebral ischemia. *A recent prospective randomized clinical evaluation of hyperventilation therapy for head injury has raised serious concern about its routine use. In this study prophylactic hyperventilation led to a worse outcome.* Hyperventilation should be used sparingly, and in general, only intermittently, to control acute increases in ICP.

Nurse head up to 20 to 35 degrees.

High-dose barbiturate therapy reduces cerebral oxygen consumption and cerebral blood flow. High-dose barbiturate therapy is an appropriate intervention for lowering ICP in those patients refractory to conventional management.

Pentobarbital is considered the drug of choice, with a loading dose of 5 to 10 mg/kg with a maintenance infusion of 1 to 3 mg/kg/hr.

Titrate to abolish the gag and cough reflex. Pentobarbital levels should be monitored and maintained between 25 and 40 mg/L.

Volume expansion and vasoactive agents are usually required to maintain MAP.

Continuous electroencephalographic monitoring is useful in monitoring the depth of barbiturate therapy.

CHAPTER 38

Guillain-Barré syndrome

DIAGNOSIS

- Clinical features

  Ascending symmetrical muscle weakness that evolves over several days to a week

  Pain and aching discomfort in muscles
  Paraesthesias
  Hypotonia with absent reflexes
  Facial diplegia common
  Autonomic dysfunction with fluctuating blood pressure and pulse, facial flushing, profuse diaphoresis

  Fisher syndrome: ophthalmoplegia, ataxia, areflexia
- CSF

  Normal pressure
  Acellular (but occasionally 10 to 50 cells found)
  Protein normal initially; but rises to reach a peak in 4 to 6 weeks
- EMG

  May be normal early in disease
  Then reduction in conduction velocity or conduction block

  Prolonged distal latencies

DIFFERENTIAL DIAGNOSIS

- Infectious mononucleosis and polyneuritis
- Hepatitis and polyneuritis
- Diphtheritic polyneuropathy
- Porphyric polyneuropathy
- Botulism
- Toxic polyneuropathies
  Triorthocresyl phosphate
  Thallium
- Lupus polyneuropathy
- Acute myasthenia gravis

TREATMENT

- Supportive

  Respiratory evaluation: frequent evaluation of respiratory function, including peak flows, forced vital capacity and respiratory reserve must be performed. A good bedside test is to see how high the patient can count on one breath—normally above 20. If the patient's peak flow, forced vital capacity, and respiratory reserve are falling, the patient should be admitted to the ICU.

  Mechanical ventilation: a rising $PaCO_2$ is a late sign of respiratory distress. A falling PaO_2 or arterial saturation is a very late sign of respiratory distress. Patients should be intubated at the first signs of dyspnea, tachypnea, or a fall in the vital capacity below 10 ml/kg.

  Prophylaxis to prevent DVT: pulmonary embolism is the commonest cause of death. Compression boots or SQ heparin is recommended. In patients who require long-term ventilation, anticoagulation with Coumadin to achieve an INR of between 1.5 and 2.5 is a practical approach.

Consider early tracheostomy in patients with severe disease

Early enteral tube feeding

Pulmonary toilet and chest physiotherapy to prevent atelectasis and pneumonia

Physical therapy to prevent flexion contractures

Regular turning to prevent decubitus ulcers

Early diagnosis and treatment of pulmonary and urinary tract infections

- Specific treatment

  Plasmapheresis: a number of large randomized trials have clearly established the usefulness of plasma exchange in the rapidly evolving phase of Guillain-Barré syndrome. Plasmapheresis instituted within 2 weeks of the onset of the disease shortens the course of the illness.

  Recently the intravenous administration of immune globulin (0.4 g/kg/day for 5 consecutive days) has been shown to be as effective as plasma exchange.

  Corticosteroids have *no beneficial* effects in patients with Guillan-Barré syndrome.

CHAPTER 39

Myasthenia gravis

Patients with myasthenia gravis may be admitted to the ICU for respiratory support or postoperatively following a thymectomy.

- Diagnosis

    Myasthenic facies: drooping eyelids, immobile mouth, snarling smile, hanging jaw in classic case

    Other signs: ptosis, diplopia, difficulty in speaking or swallowing, limb weakness

    Marked limb weakness and respiratory difficulty are seen in patients with severe disease (monitor and treat as for GBS)

    EMG and single-fiber EMG: reduction of the amplitude of compound action potentials during repetitive stimulation and blocking of single muscle fiber transmission

    Edrophonium test: increase in muscle strength after 10 mg dose (give 1 mg test dose first)

    Antibodies against the acetylcholine receptor can be demonstrated in 85% to 90% of patients

    Exclude concomitant autoimmune diseases, such as Graves disease and pernicious anemia

    Exclude botulism, which presents with diplopia, ptosis, and opthalmoparesis, with *pupils* that are usually *large and dilated*

- Management

    Anticholinesterase drugs: pyridostigmine (Mestinon) is the drug preferred by most clinicians; the dose is 15 to 90 mg q 6 hr. A *cholinergic crisis* occurs as a result of overdosing with anticholinesterase drugs and is manifest by muscarinic effects (nausea, vomiting, pallor, sweating, salivation, diarrhea, bradycardia) with increasing weakness. If the muscarinic effects are not present and weakness from pyridostigmine is suspected, the Tensilon test should be done. The weakness of a cholinergic crisis is unaffected (or worsened) by Tensilon. If the weakness improves, the patient is not receiving enough of the anticholinergic drug.

    Thymectomy is indicated in the following cases:
    All cases of thymoma
    All patients under 50 years of age who have responded poorly to anticholinesterase drugs
    A trial of steroids is indicated in patients who have responded poorly to thymectomy and anticholinesterase drugs. An initial worsening during the first 7 to 10 days may occur, necessitating close observation.

    Plasmapheresis: striking temporary remissions may be obtained by the use of plasmapheresis. This form of treatment may be lifesaving during a crisis.

DRUGS THAT INCREASE WEAKNESS IN PATIENTS WITH MYASTHENIA GRAVIS

General anesthetics
Curare
Decamethonium
Gallamine
Halothane
Methoxyflurane

Local anesthetics
Lidocaine (Xylocaine)

Antibiotics
Aminoglycoside antibiotics
  Amikacin
  Gentamicin
  Kanamycin
  Streptomycin
  Tobramycin
  Netilmicin
Bacitracin
Clindamycin
Fluoroquinolones
  Ciprofloxacin
  Norfloxacin
Tetracyclines

Antiarrhythmic drugs
Lidocaine
Procainamide
Quinidine

Antihypertensive drugs
Beta-blockers
  Atenolol
  Nadolol
  Oxprenolol
  Propranolol
  Timolol
  Metoprolol
  Acebutolol
Verapamil

Antirheumatic drugs
Chloroquine
D-penicillamine

Antiseizure drugs
Diazepam
Phenytoin
Trimethadione

Hormones
Corticosteroids and ACTH
Oral contraceptives
Thyroid hormone
Diuretics that deplete potassium

Sedatives
Barbiturates
Narcotics
Benzodiazepines
Chlorpromazine
Promazine
Phenelzine

CHAPTER 40

Neuroleptic malignant syndrome

FEATURES

- Caused by any neuroleptic agent, including piperazine, piperidine, thioxanthene, butyrophenone, and thioridazine derivatives; particularly seen with drugs that have potent antidopaminergic activity
- May occur shortly after starting the drug, after increasing the dose, or after long-term use
- Occurs in about 1% of patients treated with neuroleptic agents
- Most likely caused by central dopamine depletion
- Clinical features include the following:
    Fever, often as high as 106° F
    Altered mental status
    Tachycardia and hypertension
    Elevated creatinine phosphokinase and myoglobinuria, hypocalcemia, leukocytosis

MANAGEMENT

- Supportive therapy
- Dantrolene 0.8 to 3 mg/kg IV q 6 hr up to 10 mg/kg/ day *and*
- Bromocriptine 2.5 to 7.5 mg PO q 8 hr (1.25 to 5 mg intravaginally in women; reduces first pass hepatic metabolism)

PART SIX

INFECTIOUS DISEASES

General principles
and empiric
antibiotic protocols

GENERAL PRINCIPLES
OF ANTIMICROBIAL THERAPY

- Cultures

  Always obtain cultures before instituting antimicrobial therapy, i.e., blood, urine, and other appropriate specimens.

  At least two sets (aerobic and anaerobic) of blood cultures at two different sites should be obtained, taken a minimum of 30 minutes apart, and no more than three sets should be drawn in a 24-hour period (99% of bacteremias are diagnosed by three sets of cultures). *For optimal recovery, a minimum of 10 ml of blood should be placed in each blood culture bottle (total of 40 to 60 ml)*. Blood cultures should not be withdrawn through an arterial line (unless the line is less than 24 hours old).

  To limit contamination, venepuncture should be performed under aseptic conditions, i.e., sterile drapes should be used; the skin should be well cleansed with alcohol and Betadine; and the operator's hands should be thoroughly washed and then gloved.

  The recovery rate is very poor in patients who are currently receiving antibiotics. Patients should be off antibiotics for at least 24 hours and preferably 48 hours before culturing.

Gram stain and culture of sputum and/or tracheal aspirates are of *very little diagnostic value* in patients with suspected nosocomial or ventilator-associated pneumonia.

- When to start antibiotics

Not all patients with a fever and elevated white cell count have a bacterial or fungal infection. If no source or site of infection is obvious, and the patient is *clinically stable,* continue to culture and look for the site of infection. Antibiotics are not antipyretic agents.

Clinical signs that should prompt the institution of immediate antimicrobial therapy include the following:

Hypotension requiring volume resuscitation or inotropic support

Falling platelet count

Rising serum lactate concentration

Progressive hyperglycemia

Rising white cell count

Development of a coagulopathy, i.e., prolonged PT or PTT

All neutropenic patients with a fever should be started on antimicrobial therapy immediately after obtaining cultures.

- Narrow or broad spectrum

All neutropenic and immunocompromised patients should receive broad-spectrum cover.

Patients with *uncomplicated* community-acquired infections should receive "directed" narrow-spectrum antibiotics, e.g., patients with community-acquired urinary tract infection require narrow gram-negative cover (*E. coli*).

Patients with *complicated* community-acquired infections should receive "directed" broad-spectrum antibiotics, e.g., patients with severe community-acquired pyelonephritis require broad gram-negative cover as well as enterococcal cover.

Nursing home residents are often *colonized* with MRSA as well as resistant gram-negative bacteria. *Infections* with gram-negative bacteria are common; these patients should therefore be treated with broad-spectrum antibiotics.

- Should the spectrum be narrowed once a pathogen has been isolated?

    Data suggest that neutropenic patients should continue to receive broad-spectrum antibiotics.

    In nonneutropenic patients, the antimicrobials *must* be tailed (and narrowed) according to the sensitivities of the implicated pathogen.

- Single- or double-agent cover

    As a general rule, patients with serious gram-negative infections (suspected or proven) require double-agent cover (with additive or synergistic activity).

    The classic combination is a beta-lactam plus aminoglycoside (proven synergy in vitro and improved outcome in animal and clinical studies).

    In patients in whom an aminoglycoside is contraindicated (see Chapter 29), a double beta-lactam combination has been shown to improve outcome (combination of antipseudomonal penicillin and third generation cephalosporin or either with the monobactam aztreonam).

    Imipenem or quinolone monotherapy provides adequate antimicrobial activity *except* in patients with pseudomonas infection.

    As a general rule, patients with gram-positive infections do not require double antibiotic therapy, the only exception being enterococcal infections and patients with endocarditis.

- When to add antistaphylococcal and/or candidal cover

    Patients who have had multiple vascular procedure are at risk of staphylococcal infections (both *S. aureus* and *S. epidermidis*). These organisms are often methicillin resistant.

Antistaphylococcal therapy (vancomycin) should be started in neutropenic patients and patients with serious nosocomial sepsis who have not responded to 3 to 4 days of broad-spectrum cover.

Patients who have persistent signs of infection despite broad-spectrum and antistaphylococcal antimicrobial cover and who have risk factors for candidemia should receive antifungal therapy (see Chapter 42).

- Length of treatment
  There are no hard and fast rules.

Studies have demonstrated that in patients with gram-negative septicemia, treatment with a short course (3 days) of an aminoglycoside together with a beta-lactam is no better than a beta-lactam alone. Patients should therefore receive a full "course" of both drugs.

Patients with uncomplicated community-acquired infections should receive antibiotics for 7 to 10 days.

Patients with complicated community-acquired infections and nosocomial infections should receive antibiotics for 10 to 14 days.

Patients with *S. aureus* bacteremia should receive 4 to 6 weeks of antimicrobial therapy. Short-course therapy (2 weeks) may be associated with an unacceptably high relapse rate. Patients with methicillin-sensitive organisms have been successfully treated with high-dose oral therapy (for 4 to 6 weeks) after a few days of parenteral therapy. Recent data suggest that patients with methicillin-sensitive, right-sided endocarditis may be successfully treated with a 2-week course of a penicillinase-resistant penicillin together with gentamicin.

Patients with legionella pneumonia should receive a total of 21 days of therapy.

- Some further thoughts

  The choice of antibiotics *must* take into account the organisms (and their sensitivities) that have been isolated in your ICU and hospital. The indigenous flora differs from hospital to hospital and from unit to unit within the same hospital. The unit in which the patient becomes infected will largely determine the type of infecting organism.

  It is vitally important to track the bacteria isolated in your ICU to determine trends and outbreaks of resistant organisms.

  Rotating antibiotics may reduce the incidence of resistance to any one antibiotic.

  Third generation cephalosporins should not be used to treat *Enterobacter* infections (will induce resistance).

  In patients with renal dysfunction the half-life of aminoglycosides is increased, resulting in serum levels being elevated for a prolonged period. This enhances the renal uptake of the drug with increased nephrotoxicity. Furthermore, the dosage adjustments that are made in renal failure result in subtherapeutic and widely spaced peak levels in which a therapeutic failure can be predicted. Aminoglycoside antibiotics should therefore be avoided in patients with significant renal dysfunction.

EMPIRIC ANTIBIOTIC PROTOCOLS (BEFORE MICROBIOLOGIC DIAGNOSIS)

Meningitis

- *Adult community acquired*: cefotaxime/ceftriaxone ± ampicillin
- *Nosocomial*: ceftazidime + vancomycin ± intrathecal vancomycin; refer to Tables 41-1 and 41-2.

Table 41-1 Penetration of antimicrobials into the CSF

Penetration	Drug
Penetrates noninflamed meninges	Chloramphenicol, trimethoprim-sulfamethoxazole, isoniazid, rifampin, pyrazinamide, flucytosine, fluconazole
Penetrates to therapeutic levels in inflamed meninges	Penicillin, ampicillin, oxacillin, nafcillin, ticarcillin, piperacillin, cefuroxime, cefotaxime, ceftriaxone, ceftizoxime, ceftazidime
Unreliable penetration of meninges	Cefalothin, cefazolin, cefotetan, all amino-glycosides, vancomycin,* quinolones, ketoconazole, itraconazole, amphotericin

*Penetration of vancomycin into the CSF is erratic and unreliable. However, in some patients adequate therapeutic levels will be achieved.

Table 41-2 CSF findings according to etiology

	Bacterial	Viral	Tuberculous
Glucose mg/dl	< 40 (blood ratio < 0.4)	20-40	30-45
Protein mg/dl	100-500	50-100	100-500
WBC ($\times 10^9$/L)	1000-10,000	10-1000	100-400
Gram stain	Positive 60% to 80% untreated cases	Negative	AFB positive in up to 40%

SUSPECTED SEPTICEMIA

- Community acquired
  Aminoglycoside + third generation cephalosporin
  Ampicillin (± sulbactam) + aminoglycoside
  Quinolone
- IV drug abuser
  Vancomycin + aminoglycoside

- Febrile adult neutropenic patient
  Piperacillin (or ticarcillin) + aminoglycoside ± oxacillin

  Ceftazidime + aminoglycoside
  Imipenem ± aminoglycoside
  Aztreonam + vancomycin + aminoglycoside
- Immunocompromised or hospital acquired
  Aminoglycoside + antipseudomonal cephalosporin
  Aminoglycoside + piperacillin (or ticarcillin)
  Imipenem
  Quinolone ± aminoglycoside
  Quinolone ± aztreonam
  Antipseudomonal cephalosporin + piperacillin (or ticarcillin)

  Aztreonam + aminoglycoside

Add vancomycin for patients with multiple intravascular lines.

ENDOCARDITIS

- Native valve
  No modifying factors – penicillin G/ampicillin ± aminoglycoside

  Toxic or new valvular insufficiency – penicillin G + aminoglycoside + nafcillin/oxacillin

  IVDA – vancomycin + aminoglycoside
- Prosthetic valve
  Early—(within 3 months of surgery) – vancomycin + gentamicin + rifampin

  Late—as for native valve

BACTERIAL PERITONITIS

- Primary
  Ampicillin + aminoglycoside
  Ticarcillin/clavulanic acid

     Piperacillin/tazobactam
     Ampicillin/sulbactam
- Secondary (multiple regimens)
     Aminoglycoside + clindamycin
     Ampicillin/sulbactam ± aminoglycoside
     Ticarcillin/clavulanic acid ± aminoglycoside
     Piperacillin/tazobactam ± aminoglycoside
     Clindamycin + aztreonam
     Imipenem
     Third generation cephalosporin + metronidazole ±
     aminoglycoside
     Ampicillin + aminoglycoside + metronidazole

BILIARY TRACT INFECTION

- Piperacillin or ticarcillin ± metronidazole
- Piperacillin/tazobactam
- Ticarcillin/clavulanic acid
- Ampicillin/sulbactam
- Ampicillin + aminoglycoside + metronidazole
- Imipenem

PELVIC INFLAMMATORY DISEASE

- Ceftriaxone + doxycycline
- Ampicillin/sulbactam + doxycycline

UNCOMPLICATED PYELONEPHRITIS

- Third generation cephalosporin
- Piperacillin or ticarcillin
- Ampicillin/sulbactam
- Ampicillin + aminoglycoside

COMPLICATED PYELONEPHRITIS

- Ceftazidine
- Piperacillin/tazobactam

- Ticarcillin/clavulanic acid
- Piperacillin or ticarcillin + aminoglycoside
- Quinolone

COMMUNITY-ACQUIRED, ASPIRATION, AND NOSOCOMIAL PNEUMONIA

Refer to Chapters 9-11.

INFECTIVE ENDOCARDITIS PROPHYLAXIS

Patients at relatively high risk of endocarditis

- Prosthetic heart valves
- Previous infective endocarditis
- Cyanotic congenital heart disease
- Patent ductus arteriosus
- Aortic regurgitation
- Aortic stenosis
- Mitral regurgitation
- Mitral stenosis and regurgitation
- Ventricular septal defect
- Coarctation of the aorta
- Mitral valve prolapse with regurgitation

Procedures that require antibiotic prophylaxis

- Dental procedures, including cleaning and scaling
- Tonsillectomy and adenoidectomy
- Surgery involving gastrointestinal or upper respiratory mucosa
- Bronchoscopy with rigid bronchoscopy (not flexible bronchoscopy)
- Sclerotherapy for esophageal varices
- Esophageal dilation
- Gallbladder surgery
- Cystoscopy, urethral dilation
- Urethral catheterization if urinary tract infection is present

- Urinary tract surgery, including prostatic surgery
- Incision and drainage of infected tissue
- Vaginal hysterectomy

Antibiotic regimen

- 3 g amoxicillin 1 hour before procedure, followed by 1.5 g 6 hours later (clindamycin or erythromycin substituted for penicillin-allergic patients).
- For very high-risk patients and patients undergoing gastrointestinal or genitourinary surgery), use IV gentamicin and ampicillin or vancomycin and ampicillin.

CHAPTER 42

Nosocomial infections and infections in the immunocompromised host

Information on infections in the ICU can be found in Table 42-1 and Figs. 42-1 and 42-2.

CATHETER-ASSOCIATED SEPSIS

- Defined as bloodstream infection caused by an organism that has colonized a vascular catheter
- Incidence of catheter-related sepsis

   Approximately 1% to 5% of patients with indwelling vascular catheters will develop bloodstream infection ≈ 0.5%/catheter/day

   Increases with length in situ
   Increases with number of ports
   Increases with number of manipulations
- Colonization

   About 10% to 15% of catheters become colonized (> 15 CFU)

   Approximately 15% to 30% of colonized catheters (> 15 CFU) result in catheter sepsis
- *S. aureus* and coagulase-negative staphylococci are the most common infecting (and colonizing) organisms, followed by *Candida* species
- Replacement of a colonized catheter over a guidewire is associated with rapid colonization of the replacement catheter

Table 42-1 Spectrum of nosocomial infections in the ICU

Infection	Major pathogens	Risk factors
Urinary tract	*P. aeruginosa, Klebsiella, Enterobacter, Enterococci, S. epidermidis, Candida*	Urinary catheter, urologic manipulation, diabetes, female sex
Pneumonia	*P. aeruginosa, Acinetobacter, Klebsiella, Enterobacter, S. aureus*	Endotracheal intubation, tracheostomy, NG tube, ICP monitoring, H_2-blockers
Postsurgical/ intraabdominal sepsis	*S. aureus, E. coli* and other coliforms, enterococci, *Bacteroides fragilis*	Penetrating trauma, ruptured viscus, prolonged operation
Catheter related	Coagulase-negative staphylococci, *S. aureus*, candida	Central venous catheter > 5 days, multiport catheter, TPN
Antibiotic-associated colitis	*Clostridium difficile*	Prolonged antibiotic therapy
Candidemia	*Candida* spp.	Broad-spectrum antibiotics, central venous catheters, TPN, diabetes
Sinusitis	Often polymicrobial; *H. influenzae, pseudomonas, Acinetobacter, S. aureus*, candida, anaerobes	Nasogastric tube, nasotracheal tube, supine position

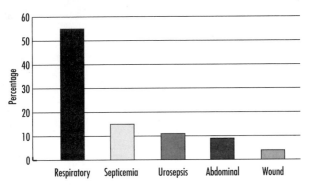

Fig. 42-1 Distribution of infections in an intensive care unit (ICU).

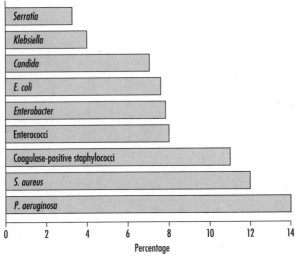

Fig. 42-2 Microbiology of nosocomial infections.

- If catheter sepsis is suspected, the catheter must be changed to a *new* site with withdrawal blood cultures and culture of the catheter tip
- Femoral catheters *are not* associated with a higher infection rate
- Incidence of catheter related sepsis is reduced by antibiotic bonded catheters
- The type of occlusive dressing and the frequency of dressing changes do affect the incidence of sepsis
- There is significant morbidity associated with line changes

RECOMMENDATIONS

- It may be prudent to follow an expectant approach, i.e., to leave the intravenous catheter in place until the following have occurred:

    Purulent discharge, cellulitis, or erythema develops at the puncture site

    Catheter malfunction

    Any positive blood cultures since the line was inserted

    Septic clinical pattern with no other obvious source of infection

    It may be wise to replace a *multilumen catheter* after 8 to 10 days even if the above criteria are not met
- All lines that are inserted in emergent situations under conditions that are not strictly aseptic should be removed within 24 hours and replaced at a new site.
- If a new catheter is replaced over a guidewire (e.g., due to catheter failure or changing type of catheter), withdrawal blood cultures and culture of the catheter tips should be done. If the blood cultures prove positive or a culture of the catheter reveals > 15 CFU, the line should be removed and inserted at a new site.

- All catheters removed from potentially septic patients should be cultured (tip and intracutaneous segment). Patients with colonized catheters (> 15 CFU) should only be treated (with appropriate antibiotics) if signs of infection do not resolve after removal of the catheter.

SINUSITIS

Nosocomial sinusitis is a common problem in ICU patients. Risk factors include nasotracheal tubes, nasogastric tubes, and patients nursed in a supine position. Almost all patients with nasotracheal tubes will develop opacification of their maxillary sinuses within 3 to 5 days of intubation. Approximately a third of these cases will prove to have infectious sinusitis. It is therefore desirable that patients in whom the length of nasotracheal intubation is expected to exceed 3 days should have all nasal tubes removed and reinserted through the mouth. The only exception would be fine-bore feeding tubes, which can be difficult to place orally.

- Diagnostic approach

  A CT scan of the paranasal sinuses should be performed in patients with a purulent nasal discharge or an offensive nasal discharge and in patients who have an undiagnosed fever with risk factors for developing sinusitis.

  Plain x-rays are of *no value* in diagnosing nosocomial sinusitis.

  Not all patients with radiologic sinusitis, i.e., opacification of the sinuses, have infectious sinusitis. Patients who have opacification of the maxillary sinuses should undergo transnasal puncture and aspiration (the nasal mucosa must be thoroughly cleaned before culture, to limit contamination). Only about 30% to 40% of patients with opacification of their maxillary sinuses will have positive cultures with purulent aspirates.

- Microbiology of nosocomial sinusitis
  Similar spectrum to that of nosocomial pneumonia
  Often polymicrobial
  Pseudomonas spp.
  Acinetobacter spp.
  S. aureus
  Candida spp.
  H. influenzae
  Anaerobes
- Treatment of infectious sinusitis
  Remove *all* nasal tubes
  Treat with broad-spectrum antibiotics, tailored to the sinus aspirate Gram stain and culture
  Local vasoconstrictors and nasal toilet

CANDIDA INFECTIONS IN THE ICU

Candida species are important opportunistic pathogens in the ICU. The Centers for Disease Control and Prevention National Nosocomial Infection Study reported that 7% of all nosocomial infections were due to candidal species. Patients with candidal infection have been shown to have a longer hospital stay and higher mortality compared with case-matched controls.

It is important to realize that *Candida* species are constituents of the normal flora found in about 30% of all healthy people. Antibiotic therapy increases the incidence of enteric colonization by up to 70%. It is probable that *most ICU patients become colonized with Candida species soon after admission. Not all patients colonized with Candida will become infected with Candida.*

- Factors predisposing patients to candida infection
  Broad-spectrum antibiotics are the single most important risk factor
  Indwelling intravenous and urinary catheters
  Parenteral alimentation
  ICU stay > 7 days
  Perforated viscus

- Clinical features

    The clinical diagnosis of systemic candidal infection is particularly difficult in the ICU patient. On the one hand the clinical picture may be indistinguishable from that of bacteremia with an acute onset of high fever, rigors, tachycardia, and hypotension. Conversely, a low-grade fever or hypothermia may be the only manifestation.

    Candida may infect the eyes causing an endophthalmitis. Funduscopy should therefore be part of the daily examination of the ICU patient.

    Although the respiratory tract is frequently colonized, invasive pulmonary candidiasis is uncommon.

    Approximately 10% of patients will present with a macular rash or discreet skin nodules.

    Other features of systemic candidiasis may include a myocarditis, meningitis, cerebral microabscesses, myositis, endocarditis, osteomyelitis, and arthritis.

- Diagnosis

    The antemortem diagnosis of systemic candidiasis is exceedingly difficult and therefore requires a high index of suspicion (an antemortem diagnosis of candidal infection is made in only 15% to 40% of patients with systemic candidiasis proven at autopsy).

    Only about 50% of patients with systemic candidiasis at postmortem have antemortem positive blood cultures.

    Serology has been shown to be of little value in the diagnosis of systemic candidiasis.

    Assays for the detection of circulating candidal antigens have a low sensitivity.

    Although candiduria may be observed in up to 80% of patients with systemic candidiasis, most patients with candiduria do not have disseminated infection or upper urinary tract infection.

An association has been demonstrated between the number of sites colonized with candida and the occurrence of invasive candidiasis in high-risk patients.

A single positive blood culture is highly predictive of candidal infection and should never be considered a contaminant.

- Management

    The initial treatment of candidal infections should include the removal of all possible foci of infection, including removal of intravascular lines and urinary catheters.

    Candidemia may resolve spontaneously after removal of an intravascular catheter. There is, however, increasing evidence that metastatic foci of infection may develop in patients who do not receive systemic antifungal therapy.

    Asymptomatic candiduria in patients with urinary catheters, in whom no suspicion exists of either renal candidiasis or renal obstruction, require change of the indwelling catheter only, plus observation. There are no data to suggest that amphotericin B bladder irrigations prevent infections in these colonized patients.

    Drainage is an integral part of the management of patients with intraabdominal suppuration in whom candida is isolated from a peritoneal culture.

    Amphotericin B has long been the standard treatment for candidemia. However, recent data suggest that fluconazole and amphotericin B may be equally efficacious in the treatment of nonneutropenic patients with candidemia.

    Amphotericin B

    A total dose of 6 to 8 mg/kg is recommended, although some authors have recommended a total dose as high as 2 grams. After a 1 mg test dose, amphotericin B is usually given in a daily dose of 0.5 mg/kg over a 2-week period. A daily dose of 1 mg/kg may be given, and this dosage is usually well tolerated. Amphotericin B should be given as an infusion in 5% dextrose water over 8 hours. Amphotericin B is associated with reversible nephrotoxicity. Fluid and sodium loading may reduce the incidence of nephrotoxicity. The dosage should not be reduced in patients with preexisting renal dysfunction because only a small fraction of the drug is excreted by the kidney.

Amphotericin B is associated with a proximal renal tubular acidosis (RTA) and a profound loss of Na^+, K^+, and Mg^{2+} in the urine. These electrolytes must be aggressively replaced.

Fever, chills, and headaches commonly occur at the initiation of therapy and are probably mediated by the release of tumor necrosis factor and interleukin-1. These side effects can be minimized by infusing the drug slowly and by premedication with antihistamines and nonsteroidal antiinflammatory agents.

Fluconazole

Loading dose: 400 mg

Maintenance dose: 200 to 400 mg as a single daily dose. The dose must be adjusted according to the calculated creatinine clearance

- Prophylaxis

  Delaying or preventing oropharyngeal, gut, and skin colonization with *Candida* species may prevent systemic infection.

  Ketoconazole has been shown to reduce the incidence of candidal infections in high-risk surgical patients.

  It is likely that fluconazole may prove to be effective in preventing infection with *Candida* species in high-risk ICU patients.

NOSOCOMIAL PNEUMONIA

Refer to Chapter 10.

CLOSTRIDIUM DIFFICILE COLITIS

C. difficile, the agent that causes pseudomembranous colitis and antibiotic-associated diarrhea, has become a common nosocomial pathogen. *C. difficile* is responsible for virtually all cases of pseudomembranous colitis and for up to 20% of cases of antibiotic-associated diarrhea without colitis. The spores of *C. difficile* are easily transmitted by the oral-fecal route from one patient to the next and may become widely disseminated throughout a hospital. Although reported in the preantibiotic era, antibiotics are the most important risk factor leading to colonization and colitis. The normal colonic flora resists colonization by *C. difficile*; however, broad-spectrum antibiotics with activity against enteric bacteria disrupt the normal flora, allowing colonization. Approximately 25% of hospitalized adults recently treated with antibiotics will become colonized with *C. difficile*. Once established in the colon, pathogenetic strains of *C. difficile* produce two exotoxins (toxin A and B) that cause diarrhea and colitis.

Antimicrobial agents that induce *C. difficile*

- Frequent induction
  - Ampicillin and amoxicillin
  - Cephalosporins
  - Clindamycin
- Infrequent induction
  - Tetracyclines
  - Sulphanomides
  - Erythromycin
  - Chloramphenicol
  - Trimethoprim
  - Quinolones

- Rare or no induction
    Parenteral aminoglycosides
    Metronidazole
    Vancomycin

The majority of hospital patients infected with *Clostridium difficile* are asymptomatic. *C. difficile* infection commonly presents as diarrhea that is mild to moderate, sometimes accompanied by lower abdominal cramping. Symptoms usually begin during or shortly after antibiotic therapy but are occasionally delayed for several weeks. Severe colitis without pseudomembrane formation may occur with profuse, debilitating diarrhea, abdominal pain, and distension. Common systemic manifestations include fever, nausea, anorexia, and malaise. A neutrophilia and increased numbers of fecal leukocytes are common. Pseudomembranous colitis is the most dramatic manifestation of *C. difficile infection*; these patients have marked abdominal and systemic signs and symptoms and may develop a fulminant and life-threatening colitis. The diagnosis of *C. difficile* infection is made by the demonstration of *C. difficile* toxins in the stool, using the stool cytotoxin test.

Management

Treatment of asymptomatic carriers is not recommended. The first step in managing patients is to discontinue antibiotic therapy, if possible. Patients with mild diarrhea may not require any other treatment. However, in the ICU this is often not possible, and therefore specific therapy aimed at eradicating *C. difficile* is necessary. Oral metronidazole (250 mg q 6 hr) is the drug of first choice. Oral vancomycin (125 mg q 6 hr) is reserved for patients who cannot tolerate or who do not have a response to metronidazole. Patients who cannot tolerate oral medication can be treated with intravenous metronidazole. In general, sigmoidoscopy should be avoided in severe colitis because of the risk of perforation.

ACALCULOUS CHOLECYSTITIS

Acalculous cholecystitis, although relatively uncommon, is an important infection in critically ill patients. It is often unrecognized and is therefore potentially life threatening. Only about 10% of cases of acute cholecystitis in the ICU are associated with gallstones, which are usually considered an incidental finding rather than the cause. Critically ill patients have multiple factors that increase their risk for developing this complication.

The diagnosis of acalculous cholecystitis is often exceedingly difficult and requires a high index of suspicion. Pain in the right upper quadrant is the finding that most often leads the clinician to the correct diagnosis, but it may frequently be absent. Nausea, vomiting, and fever are other associated clinical features. The clinical findings and laboratory workup in patients with acalculous cholecystitis are, however, often nonspecific. The most difficult patients are those recovering from abdominal sepsis who deteriorate again, misleadingly suggesting a flare-up of the original infection.

Radiologic investigations are required for a presumptive diagnosis. Ultrasound is the most common radiologic investigation used in the diagnosis of acalculous cholecystitis, with a sensitivity and specificity of greater than 80% and 90% respectively (features include increased wall thickness, intramural lucencies, gallbladder distension, pericholecystic fluid, and intramural sludge). In ICU patients, hepatobiliary scintigraphy has a high false-positive rate (> 50%), limiting the value of this test. However, a normal scan virtually excludes acalculous cholecystitis. CT scanning has been reported to have a high sensitivity and specificity.

Management

Once the presumptive diagnosis has been made, the management consists of both medical and interventional therapies. The gallbladder either needs to be drained or removed surgically. Percutaneous cholecystomy is usually the initial procedure of choice, with interval cholecystomy performed when (and if) the patient is considered a suitable surgical candidate. It should be noted that acalculous cholecystitis is primarily a noninfectious disease, with bacterial invasion being a secondary event (at least a third of patients have sterile bile). However, antibiotics with adequate gram-negative coverage are usually prescribed.

PYREXIA IN THE ICU

Refer to Fig. 42-3.

PATHOGENS IN IMMUNOCOMPROMISED PATIENTS

Granulocytopenic

- Bacteria
    Gram negative
        Escherichia coli
        Klebsiella pneumoniae
        Pseudomonas aeruginosa
        Enterobacter spp.
        Acinetobacter spp.
    Gram positive
        Staphylococcus epidermidis

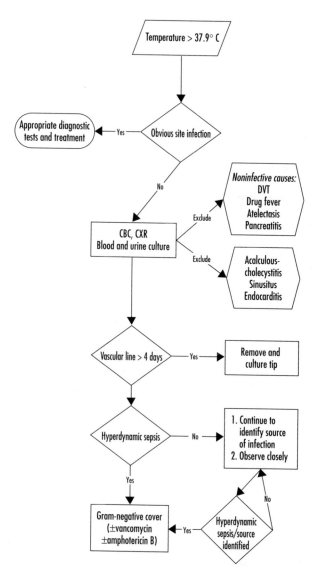

Fig. 42-3 Pyrexia in an intensive care unit (ICU).

CHAPTER 43

HIV infection

As a consequence of antimicrobial prophylaxis (especially against PCP) and changes in the epidemiology and treatment of HIV-associated illness, the spectrum of diseases requiring intensive care has changed. PCP remains the commonest reason for admission to the ICU; however, other causes of respiratory failure as well as many other conditions account for any increasing number of ICU admissions. The patient's general physiologic condition and nutritional status are important factors in determining outcome. Only patients who are likely to derive a benefit from intensive care warrant admission to an ICU.

In the early part of the AIDS epidemic, most admissions were due to respiratory failure caused by PCP. From 1980 to 1987, the mortality rate of patients with PCP who required mechanical ventilation was approximately 85%. With the adjunctive use of high-dose corticosteroid therapy, the mortality has been reduced to between 40% and 60%.

HIV CLASSIFICATION SYSTEM

Refer to Table 43-1.

- Category B symptoms
    Thrush
    Oral hairy leukoplakia
    Zoster, multidermatomal or recurrent

Constitutional symptoms
Vaginal or vulval candidiasis
Cervical dysplasia
Pelvic inflammatory disease
Immune thrombocytopenic purpura
Peripheral neuropathy
Bacillary angiomatosis
Listeriosis
Nocardiosis
- Category C symptoms
Candidiasis, esophageal
Cervical cancer
Coccidioidomycosis
Cryptosporidiosis
Cytomegalovirus disease (other than liver, spleen, or nodes)

Encephalopathy, HIV related
Herpes simplex: chronic mucocutaneous, bronchitic, pneumonia, or esophatigis

Histoplasmosis
Isosporiasis
Kaposi sarcoma
Lymphoma: Burkitt, or primary, brain
Mycobacterium avium complex

Table 43-1 Stages of HIV disease

CD4 T-cell category (cells/μl³)	Asymptomatic category A	Symptomatic category B	AIDS indicator condition (category C)
> 500	A1	B1	C1
200-499	A2	B2	C2
< 200	A3	B3	C3

Shaded area refers to diagnosis of AIDS.

Mycobacterium tuberculosis
Mycobacterium, other
Pneumocystis carinii pneumonia
Pneumonia, recurrent
Progressive multifocal leukoencephalopathy
Salmonella septicemia, recurrent
Toxoplasmosis of brain
Wasting syndrome caused by HIV (> 10% body weight)

COURSE OF HIV INFECTION

Refer to Table 43-2 and Fig. 43-1.

Table 43-2 Infections in the HIV-positive patient

Type	Transition	Late
Parasites/protozoa	*Strongyloides* *Giardia lamblia* *Entamoeba histolytica*	*Isospora belli* *Cryptosporidium* *Microsporidia*
Mycobacterium	Typical TB	Disseminated MTB and MAC
Bacteria	*S. pneumoniae,* *H. influenzae,* *S. aureus* *Legionella* sp.	Transition organisms and *Rhodococcus equi*
Fungi	Oral and vaginal Candidiasis	*Pneumocystis carinii* *Cryptococcus* Histoplasmosis Aspergillosis Esophageal candidiasis
Viruses	HSV	VZV and CMV
Malignant	Kaposi sarcoma	Lymphoma
Neurologic disease	Neurovascular syphilis	Dementia, mass lesions

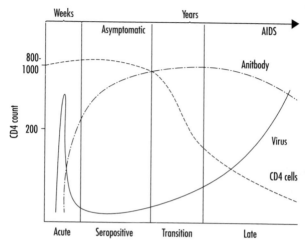

Fig. 43-1 Course of HIV infection.

OUTLINE OF HIV MANAGEMENT

Refer to Table 43-3.

- CD4 200 to 500

    Consider antiretroviral therapy, especially if symptomatic
- CD4 < 200

    Antiretroviral therapy

    PCP prophylaxis

    Fungal prophylaxis if previous cryptococcus infection

    Toxoplasma prophylaxis if previous toxoplasma infection
- CD4 < 100

    ? MAC prophylaxis with rifabutin

TREATMENT OF *PNEUMOCYSTIS CARINII* PNEUMONIA

- The following are two "accepted" management approaches for the HIV-positive patient with suspected PCP:

Table 43-3 Indications, contraindications, and dosages for antiretroviral drugs

Indication/contra-indication/dosage	Zidovidine (AZT)	Didanosine (DDI)	Zalcitabine (DDC)
Indicated for	HIV CNS disease, thrombocytopenia CD4 < 200, ? < 500	Anemia, neutropenia, AZT failure	Anemia, neutropenia, AZT failure
Relative contraindication	Hg 8-9.5 ANC 750-1000	Inactive alcoholism IV pentamidine therapy, mod PN increased amylase, seizures	Moderate PN
Strong contraindication	Transfusion-dependent anemia ANC < 500-750	History of pancreatitis active alcoholism, severe PN	Severe PN
Major adverse effects	Bone marrow supression, myopathy	Pancreatitis, PN, ? seizures	PN
Dosage	200 mg tid	Based on weight and CD4 count*	0.375-0.75 tid

PN, Peripheral neuropathy; ANC, absolute neutrophil count.

*CD4 > 50   CD4 < 50

WT > 60 kg: 200 mg bid   WT > 60 kg: 100 mg bid

WT < 60 kg: 125 mg bid   WT < 60 kg: 75 mg bid

To perform bronchoscopy on all patients (who have negative induced sputum)

To treat patients empirically for PCP and perform bronchoscopy and BAL in those patients whose condition does not improve within 3 days of therapy

- Antimicrobial therapy

    Trimethoprim-sulfamethoxazole 20 mg/kg/day (of trimethoprim) in four divided doses. Usually start IV; switch to same oral dose when patient starts to improve for a total of 21 days

    Pentamidine 4 mg/kg/day (as an 8-hour infusion) daily for a total of 21 days

    Dapsone 50 mg PO bid *plus* trimethoprim 20 mg/kg/day in divided doses for 21 days

    Clindamycin 600 to 900 mg IV q 8 hr *plus* primaquine 15 to 30 mg PO OD

- If Pao_2 < 70 mm Hg (on room air), add prednisone 40 mg q 12 hr for 5 days, then 40 mg qd for 5 days, then 20 mg qd for 11 days.
- *Treatment failure*: average time to improvement is 7 to 10 days, and there is often clinical and radiologic worsening over the first 3 to 4 days of therapy. If there is failure to improve or clinical worsening by 7 to 10 days, switching drugs can be done, but it is helpful in only a minority of cases. Thus it appears that drug resistance is rarely the problem; the cause of treatment failure is more likely host failure.
- *Mechanical ventilation*: mechanical ventilation is a reasonable consideration for the first episode of pneumocystis in relatively well-nourished patients who are agreeable; as many as 40% of patients are successfully weaned off the ventilator. Mechanical ventilation should be avoided in patients with multiple episodes and patients with advanced disease, since the likelihood of survival is low.

TREATMENT OF TOXOPLASMOSIS

Empiric therapy for presumptive cerebral toxoplasmosis should be used only for cases of typical toxoplasmosis. If features are atypical for toxoplasmosis, it is best to obtain a brain biopsy if aggressive therapy is desired. Atypical features include the following:

- Single lesion on MRI IgG
- Absence of serum lgG toxoplasma antibodies
- No contrast enhancement

Treatment

- Sulfadiazine 1 to 2 g PO q 6 hr *plus* pyrimethamine 100 mg PO loading dose, then 50 mg PO daily
- Clindamycin 600 to 1200 mg IV or 600 mg PO q 6 hr *plus* pyrimethamine 100 mg PO loading dose, then 50 mg PO daily

Suppression therapy (lifelong)

- Sulfadiazine and pyrimethamine in half treatment dose
- Fansidar
- Clindamycin and pyrimethamine

CRYPTOSPORIDIUM

- Opiate-derived antimotility agents
- Octreotide 50 to 200 μg SQ tid (very expensive)

CRYPTOCOCCUS

Current data suggest that amphotericin B may be more effective in bringing the acute disease under control, while fluconazole may be more effective in chronic suppression once initial therapy has sterilized the CSF.

- *Amphotericin B* (± *flucytosine*): start with high dose of 0.7 to 1.0 mg/kg IV for 2 to 4 weeks, then switch to fluconazole
- *Fluconazole*: may be used initially in less ill patients; dose of 400 mg/day PO

MYCOBACTERIUM AVIUM-INTRACELLULAR COMPLEX

In general, when AFB smears are positive, or there is growth of mycobacterium, patients should be started on drugs effective for myocbacterium tuberculosis with or without MAC coverage until the species of AFB has been identified, or *M. tuberculosis* is ruled out. However, AFB in the blood or stool are usually MAC, whereas respiratory or lymph node AFB could be MAC or *M. tuberculosis*. MAC cultured from the sputum or stool may not represent disseminated MAC, and it may not be necessary to treat the patient at this stage of the disease.

Suggested initial regimen

- Clarithromycin 500 mg PO bid *plus*
- Ethambutol 20 mg/kg/day *and*
- Rifabutin 600 mg/day PO *or*
- Clofazimine 100 mg/day PO

HERPES SIMPLEX

Acyclovir 200 to 800 mg PO 5 times per day for ulcerative mucocutaneous lesions

CYTOMEGALOVIRUS

Therapy is given for potentially life- or sight-threatening CMV and *not* just positive CMV antibodies or positive culture from urine or bronchoscopy. Indications for therapy are as follows:

- Retinitis
- Gastrointestinal—enterocolitis, esophagitis, gastritis
- Pneumonia (proven by lung biopsy)

Treatment

- *Gancyclovir*: 5 mg/kg IV over 1 hour q 12 for 2 to 4 weeks. Do not use if absolute neutrophil count is less than 500. Adjust dose according to renal function.
- *Foscarnet*: Drug is nephrotoxic and dose is based on accurate calcuation of creatinine clearance.

Sepsis syndrome and septic shock

Sepsis and septic shock are heterogenous clinical syndromes that can be triggered by many microorganisms, including gram-negative bacteria, gram-positive bacteria, and fungi. The sepsis syndrome is characterized as the systemic response to infection manifested by tachycardia, tachypnea, alteration in temperature, and leukopenia or leukocytosis. Septic shock is defined as severe sepsis accompanied by hypotension (MAP < 60 mm Hg).

COMMON CLINICAL MANIFESTATIONS OF SEPSIS

- Fever and hypothermia
- Tachycardia
- Tachypnea
- Altered mental status
- Coma
- Respiratory alkalosis
- Metabolic acidosis and lactic acidosis
- Thrombocytopenia
- Consumptive coagulopathy
- Neutrophilia and neutropenia
- Acute lung injury and ARDS
- Proteinuria
- Acute tubular necrosis
- Intrahepatic cholestasis

- Elevated transaminases
- Hyperglycemia
- Hypoglycemia

PATHOPHYSIOLOGY OF SEPSIS

As can be seen from Table 44-1, the processing of microbial antigens results in the release of an enormous number of primary, secondary, and tertiary mediators that interact in an exceedingly complex manner, the end result being the sepsis syndrome. On the one hand this process may rid the host of the infecting microbe, on the other it may result in the death of the host. It is likely that the uncontrolled activation of the cascading network of mediators leads to septic shock and death.

Hematologic manifestations of sepsis

The hematologic manifestations of sepsis are highlighted as they play a major role in the septic process.

The neutrophil

Inflammatory mediators result in a brisk increase in polymorphonuclear production and release from the bone marrow, resulting in a leukocytosis with "left shift." Peripheral blood smears frequently reveal hypersegmented polymorphonuclear leukocytes and band or immature forms of polymorphonuclear leukocytes. Typically there is evidence of toxic granulation (increased number of leukocyte granules), vacuolization, and Dohle bodies.

Neutrophils play a major role in mediating endothelial damage and tissue injury in sepsis. Inflammatory mediators, such as C3a, C5a, NO activate neutrophils, result in an increase in primary and secondary granules and expression of surface adhesion molecules (e.g., integrins). Cytokines such as TNF-α result in the up regulation of endothelial adhesion molecules. Irreversible binding of neutrophils with endothelial adhesion molecules ensues. This process leads to neutrophil adhesion, diapedesis and degranulation with bacterial (and tissue) injury. It must be emphasized that the circulating pool of neutrophils represents a small fraction of the total neutrophil pool both in health and during sepsis. In patients with "overwhelming sepsis" it is not uncommon for the patient to present with a neutropenia. *The neutropenia of sepsis must be distinguished from the neutropenia associated with chemotherapeutic agents and that caused by marrow infiltration.* Patients with septic neutropenia almost always have a hypercellular marrow (sepsis-induced bone marrow failure is uncommon) and *an increased neutrophil pool.* The neutropenia in these patients is almost certainly due to the accumulation of neutrophils in the microcapillary beds and tissues of the inflamed organs. In patients with sepsis-associated neutropenia the neutrophil count usually rises within 24 to 48 hours of initiating antibiotic (and other supportive) therapy.

The clotting cascade (also see Chapter 54)

As is outlined below, sepsis activates the coagulation cascade by a number of complex interacting mechanisms. The net result being microvascular thrombosis, consumption of coagulation factors, with a bleeding tendency (DIC).

- *Endotoxin*: activates factor XII
- *Platelet activating factor (PAF)*: increased synthesis of thromboxane B_2 and PGE_2
- TNF

    Increased expression of cell surface tissue factor and activation of the contact system

    Generation of thrombin
    Decreases thrombomodulin expression and therefore activation of protein C

    Induction of plasminogen activator inhibitor
    Suppression of tissue type plasminogen activator

Table 44-1 The "sepsis cascade"

Bacterial products	Antigen processing	Mediators	Clinical result
Endotoxin	Monocytes	TNF-α	Endothelial damage
Peptidoglycan	Macrophages	IL-1	Capillary permeability
Mennan (fungal wall)	Lymphocytes	IL-2	Endothelial swelling
Exotoxins		IL-6	Peripheral vasodilation
		IL-8	Maldistribution of blood flow
		C3a, C5a	Myocardial depression
		Endorphins	Intravascular coagulation
		O⁻ radicals	Hyperdynamic syndrome
		PAF	Organ dysfunction
		Kinins	Tissue necrosis
		Interferons	Cellular dysoxia
		Nitric oxide	Stress ulceration
		Histamine	Hepatic dysfunction

Prostaglandins	Bowel mucosal ischemia
Leukotrienes	Bacterial translocation
WBCs	Encephalopathy
Integrins	Polyneuropathy
Selectins	Insulin resistance
ICAMs	MSOF
Renin-angiotensin	
Endothelin	
Coagulation factors	
Fibrinolytic system	
Colony stimulating factors	
Transforming growth factor	
Endotoxin binding protein	

MANAGEMENT OF THE SEPTIC PATIENT

As can be seen from Table 44-1, the sepsis syndrome is the end result of the complex interaction of a myriad of primary, secondary, and tertiary mediators. Furthermore, it should be obvious that once the patient has manifested signs and symptoms of sepsis, interference (immunomodulation) of one (or a number) of these inflammatory mediators is unlikely to profoundly impact upon the clinical course of sepsis. In addition, the further established the septic process, the less impact immunomodulation is likely to have. Table 44-2 summarizes the results of those studies that have attempted immunomodulation in septic patients.

It is possible that immunomodulating agents may impair host defense mechanism and be detrimental to patients. Anti-TNF and anti-IL-1 agents have not been shown to improve outcome in the treatment of human sepsis, and in fact septic shock may be potentially harmful. The identification of patients in whom an exaggerated cytokine response develops and who are thus likely to benefit from antiinflammatory treatment strategies remains an important issue. The timing, duration, and delivery of these therapies to tissue compartments are other critical unresolved issues.

The cornerstone of the management of patients with sepsis remains antibiotic therapy, the surgical drainage of pus, and supportive therapy. Hemodynamic support is particularly important in septic patients. Most septic patients demonstrate some degree of peripheral vasodilation and myocardial depression. Although contractility is depressed, most patients have a hyperdynamic circulation with a high cardiac index. This hemodynamic pattern is largely due to peripheral vasodilation, which is present in almost all septic patients (except in some preterminal patients). Less than 10% of septic patients have severe myocardial depression with sepsis-induced cardiogenic shock. The support of patients with sepsis and septic shock incorporates many of the principles involved in the management of patients with ARDS (see Chapter 5).

The following approach to hemodynamic support is suggested:

- Volume replacement remains the first line of hemo-dynamic support (see Chapters 5, 14, and 15).
- Pulmonary artery catheterization is recommended in patients who remain hypotensive after 1.5 to 2 L of volume replacement and/or have evidence of tissue hypoxemia and/or who develop worsening gas exchange with volume replacement.
- Titrate fluid replacement to maintain the PCWP 10 to 12 mm Hg (avoid overresuscitation).
- Recent clinical data suggest that *norepinephrine* may be the vasocative agent of choice in hyperdynamic sepsis. High-dose dopamine should be avoided. Low-dose dopamine (2 µg/kg/min) may have a role in patients who remain oliguric despite an adequate mean arterial pressure.
- Dobutamine should be used in patients with myocar-dial depression caused by sepsis or underlying myo-cardial disease.
- The hemodynamic profile should be titrated to maintain a mean arterial pressure > 70 mm Hg and to achieve adequate tissue oxygenation (see Chapter 53).
- Hemodynamic manipulation to achieve predeter-mined, patient independent hemodynamic goals can-not be recommended. Recent data suggest that such an approach may increase mortality.

Table 44-2 Immunomodulation therapy in sepsis

Type of immuno-modulation	Agent(s) used	Outcome
Corticosteroids	Methylprednisolone	No clinical benefit increased complications
Pentoxifylline		No good clinical data
Thromboxane and leukotriene antagonists	Ibuprofen, thromboxane, and leuko-triene receptor antagonists	No clinical benefit animal data only
Antioxidants	Superoxide dismutase, vitamin E, allopurinol	No good clinical data
Plasma exchange	CAVH, CAVHD	No clinical benefit (? worse outcome)
Antiendotoxin antibodies	J5 antiserum, E5 (murine IgM), HA-1A (human IgM)	No clinical benefit (? worse outcome)
Endotoxin neutralizing protein	Recombinant protein	Animal data only

Anti-TNF antibodies	Murine monoclonal antibody	No clinical benefit
TNF receptor	Recombinant human TNF receptor antagonist	No clinical benefit (? worse outcome)
IL-1 antagonists	Recombinant IL-1 receptor antagonist	No clinical benefit
Leukocyte CD11/18 adhesion complex	CD11/18 monoclonal antibody	Increased mortality in animal studies
Increasing circulating neutrophils	Recombinant granulocyte colony-stimulating factor	Animal data only
Nitric oxide synthetase	N-methyl-L-arginine (L-NMA) methylene blue	Animal data only ? short-term clinical benefit
Platelet activating factor	?	?

PART SEVEN

MISCELLANEOUS ICU TOPICS

CHAPTER 45

ICU admission criteria and ICU organization

The technologic advances that medicine has witnessed in the last few decades are no more apparent than in the ICU. Yet, when used inappropriately, this technology may not save lives or improve the quality of life, but rather may transform death into a prolonged, miserable, and undignified process. Life support technology is intended to provide temporary support for patients with potentially reversible organ failure and is not a measure to conquer death.

Data suggest that many patients with non–life-threatening illnesses are admitted to intensive care units. These patients are admitted for monitoring because their physicians feel "uncomfortable" managing them in a non-ICU setting. Such patients represent an abuse of a limited resource, often delaying or preventing the admission of patients more likely to benefit from ICU care. It is therefore important that all potential admissions to the ICU be screened to ensure that the patients are likely to benefit from being admitted to the ICU. The intensivist is that person best qualified to act as the gatekeeper of the ICU.

ADMISSION CRITERIA: GENERAL PRINCIPLES

Patients who may potentially benefit from admission to an ICU can be stratified into high- and low-priority patients.

High-priority patients

These are critically ill, unstable patients who have acute potentially reversible conditions and require intensive treatments (such as ventilator support and vasoactive drug therapy) and close continuous observation. When the reversibility and prognosis of a patient's condition is uncertain, a "time-limited" therapeutic trial in the ICU may be justified. This category excludes poorly functioning patients with chronic underlying diseases and patients with terminal illnesses.

Low-priority patients

This category includes patients at "risk" of requiring intensive treatment and patients with severe, disabling, and irreversible medical conditions.

Patients with advanced chronic disease, patients with terminal illnesses, and patients who have suffered a catastrophic insult should only be admitted to an ICU if there is a chance that the patient may benefit from aggressive management in an ICU *and* the patient or surrogate is prepared to accept the burden that such therapy may incur.

SPECIFIC ICU ADMISSION CRITERIA

The size, type, and referral base of a hospital, as well as the number of ICU beds, largely determines the selection criteria for admission to a hospital ICU. ICU bed availability has a large impact on admission criteria. ICU beds account for 8% of all acute care beds in the United States. This compares with between 1% and 2% in other western nations. Consequently, ICU patients in the United States have a lower acuity of illness and a higher mean age, with a larger proportion of patients being admitted for monitoring alone, compared with other industrialized countries.

The merits of each potential ICU admission should be assessed on an individual basis, taking into account the patient's premorbid condition, nature, and severity of the acute illness, benefits to be gained from admission to an ICU, as well as any advance directives. These factors must be balanced against the availability of ICU beds to ensure the most appropriate use of a limited and very costly resource. Poor or inadequate care on the "floor" is not an appropriate reason for admission to an ICU.

The following serve as *guidelines* in selecting patients who are most likely to benefit from the physiologic support provided in an ICU:

Physiologic indications

- Systolic BP < 90 mm Hg and/or drop in systolic BP of > 20 mm Hg after 1000 ml of fluid resuscitation
- Inotropic agents required to maintain blood pressure and tissue perfusion
- Diastolic blood pressure > 120 mm Hg *and* one of the following:
  Pulmonary edema
  Hypertensive encephalopathy
  Dissecting aortic aneurysm
  Acute myocardial ischemia
  Preeclampsia or eclampsia (diastolic > 110 mm Hg)
  Subarachnoid hemorrhage (diastolic > 100 mm Hg)
- Sinus tachycardia
  > 130/min (age < 50 years)
  > 120/min (age > 50 years)
- Respiratory rate > 30 min
- Pao_2 < 55 mm Hg with Fio_2 ≥ 0.4
- Arterial pH < 7.20 (ketoacidosis < 7.10)
- Temperature < 32° C
- Hyperkalemia, with serum K^+ > 6 mEq/L
- Glasgow coma score < 12 following:
  Head trauma
  Seizures

Metabolic derangements
Subarachnoid hemorrhage
Drug overdose
Excluding, cerebrovascular accidents

Disease-specific indications for common ICU admitting diagnoses

NOTE: These indications are in addition to the physiologic indications listed above.

- Pneumonia (one physiologic factor or two of the following factors:)

  $30 < WBC < 4 \times 10^9/L$

  $BUN > 20$ mg/dl

  $PaO_2 < 60$ mm Hg (room air)

  Multilobe involvement

  Platelet $< 80\ 000 \times 10^9/l$

  Confusion
- Asthma

  Difficulty talking because of breathlessness

  Altered level of consciousness

  FEV1 and/or peak flow < 40% predicted

  Pulsus paradoxus > 18 mm Hg

  Pneumothorax or pneumomediastinum

  $PaO_2 < 65$ mm Hg on 40% O_2

  $PaCO_2 > 40$ mm Hg

  Patient "tiring"
- COPD

  Acute respiratory acidosis with pH < 7.25

  Altered mental status

  Pneumothorax or pneumomediastinum

  Patient "tiring"
- Myocardial ischemia

  Unstable angina

  All but "small" acute myocardial infarctions presenting within 24 hours of chest pain

All complicated acute myocardial infarctions (Patients admitted to hospital to "rule out" AMI do not gain any benefit from being admitted to an ICU)

- GI bleeding

  Ongoing, persistent bleeding, or rebleeding

  Hemodynamic instability (systolic BP < 90 mm Hg, pulse rate > 120/min) or postural changes in blood pressure and pulse after 1000 ml of fluid resuscitation

  Massive bleed: defined as a loss of 30% or more of estimated blood volume or bleeding requiring blood transfusion of six or more units/24 hours

- Pancreatitis

  Three or more Ranson criteria

- Preoperative optimization (pulmonary artery catheterization)

  AMI within 6 months

  Major noncardiac surgery and NYHA grade III or IV cardiac failure and/or ejection fraction of < 40%

  Major vascular surgery

- Postoperative care

  AMI within 6 months

  Major noncardiac surgery and NYHA grade III or IV cardiac failure and/or ejection fraction of < 40%

  Major vascular surgery
  Major cardiothoracic surgery

  COPD patients with preoperative FEV1 < 2 L and/or $Paco_2$ > 45 mm Hg undergoing major surgery

  Morbidly obese patients

- Trauma

  Major polytrauma
  Major thoracic injury
  Head injury with GCS < 12

- Burns
    - Adults > 25% BSA
    - Children > 20% BSA
    - Full-thickness burns > 10% BSA
    - Burns of face, hands, feet, eyes, ears, or perineum
    - High-voltage electric injury
    - Inhalation injury or associated trauma

    Medical conditions that increase the patient's medical risk

ICU ORGANIZATIONAL STRUCTURE

The organizational structure of an ICU has an enormous impact on the quality of care delivered and patient outcome. Open units are those in which admission of patients to the ICU is uncontrolled and management of the patients is at the discretion of each private attending physician. Admissions are based on a first-come, first-served basis. The role of the intensivist in an open unit is to attempt to achieve a balance among all the consultants involved in the care of the critically ill patient, and to attempt to prevent the patient from "falling through the cracks" because of the fractionated care. Critical care, however, is among the most labor intensive of all specialities, requiring long hours at the bedside, with frequent and repeated evaluations of the patient. This is impossible for even the most dedicated private practitioners or surgeons to achieve since most of their time is spent in their offices or operating rooms. Consequently, the private physician "portions off" the patients' care to a number of organ-specific subspecialists (known as the *SODs*, or *single organ doctors*). This frequently results in conflicting treatment strategies. Furthermore, both accountability and responsibility are also portioned off, with no physician assuming ultimate responsibility for the patients' care. Such a system is highly cost-inefficient and not conducive to achieving optimal patient care.

Closed units are those in which the intensivist screens all admissions and discharges and assumes full responsibility for all aspects of the patients' care. The closed ICU is a highly structured and controlled environment. Intensivists are available 24 hours a day to provide care at the bedside. In critical care, it is the intensive attention at the bedside that makes the difference between living and dying. Critical care cannot be practiced from conference rooms or remotely by telephone. It is my opinion that ICU patients are best managed by dedicated full-time intensivists (who have no competing obligations) who have undergone specialized *clinical training* to provide them with the necessary knowledge, skills, and attitudes required to achieve the best outcome for the critically ill and injured patient.

Do-not-resuscitate orders and withdrawal of life support

DO-NOT-RESUSCITATE ORDERS

Cardiopulmonary resuscitation (CPR) is a common medical procedure performed on most patients who die in hospital. The Presidents Commission for the Study of Ethical Problems in Medicine and Biomedical Research has stated that "a specific instruction is necessary if CPR is not to be instituted." Consequently, the current policy in most hospitals in the United States is to perform CPR on all patients who die, unless the patient or his or her surrogate or medical power of attorney has issued an instruction for this procedure not to be performed. However, approximately only one in every ten patients who undergoes CPR will survive to hospital discharge, and this success rate has remained largely unchanged over the last decade, despite the widespread use of do-not-resuscitate orders.

Closed-chest massage, as first described by Kouwenhoven in 1960, was intended primarily to be administered to otherwise "healthy patients" with reversible conditions who experienced a sudden and unexpected cardiorespiratory arrest. A monograph on CPR written in 1965 states that CPR is intended to "resuscitate the victims of an acute insult, whether it be from drowning, electrical shock, untoward effects of drugs, anesthetic accident, heart block, acute myocardial infarction, or surgery" (Talbott JH et al: *Fundamentals of cardiopulmonary resuscitation*, Philadelphia, 1965, F. A. Davis.) At present, however, it is the current practice to attempt CPR on any patient who dies, regardless of the underlying illness, except in those circumstances where a DNR order exists. Cardiac resuscitation when applied to critically ill patients may restore cardiac function, but it does not prevent death, rather it prolongs the dying process.

The American College of Chest Physicians (ACCP), the Society of Critical Care Medicine (SCCM), and the American Thoracic Society (ATS) have issued consensus statements endorsing the concept that physicians are not obligated to provide life-supporting interventions that are futile. An intervention was defined as being futile if reasoning and experience indicate that the intervention would be highly unlikely to result in a meaningful survival for that patient.

If it is judged that the patient would not benefit from performing CPR, should he or she suffer a cardiac arrest, then, as with other forms of medical therapy, where there is a certainty that the intervention will not be of benefit to the patient, it should not be offered. However (according to the policy of most hospitals in the United States), the family or patient *must* be informed of the futility of CPR and agree with the decision not to provide futile care (including CPR). Furthermore, the order *must* be written in the patient's medical record together with a summary of the discussion held with the family.

It should be noted that a DNR order does not preclude a patient from being admitted to an ICU or undergoing an operation. Furthermore, a DNR order does not imply that a patient's treatment should be limited in any way. It is simply an order which states that "chest compressions will not be performed, ACLS drugs will not be given, and the patient will not be intubated should he suffer a cardiac or respiratory arrest." Patients with DNR orders undergoing surgery, should have the DNR order reversed during the period of surgery.

WITHHOLDING AND WITHDRAWAL
OF LIFE SUPPORT

In the past few decades medicine has made tremendous technologic advances. Yet, when used inappropriately, these innovations may not improve the quality of life but rather prolong the dying process. The vast armamentarium of technologic gadgetry at the disposal of the modern physician has allowed him or her to change the dying process. Most Americans die in the hospital, often with heroic measures being taken to prevent their death. Yet research has shown that most dying patients would prefer to die at home.

According to Hippocrates, the purpose of medicine is "to do away with the suffering of the sick, to lessen the violence of their diseases, and to refuse to treat those who are overmastered by their diseases, realizing that in such cases, medicine is powerless." The ethical principles of beneficence (being of benefit to the patient) and nonmaleficence (doing no harm) underlie the modern practice of medicine. Life-sustaining interventions should not have as their sole goal the unqualified prolongation of a patient's biologic life; instead, the goal should be to restore and maintain a patient's well-being.

A physician has no ethical obligation to provide a life-sustaining intervention that is judged to be futile. Should a physician decide to withhold or withdraw life-sustaining therapeutic interventions, the physician must tell the patient or the surrogate of this decision and explain the rationale. The physician must, however, continue to give all other medical care necessary to provide comfort for the patient. Should the patient or surrogate disagree with this decision, the physician has the option of tranferring the care of the patient to another physician who is willing to abide by the patient's (surrogate's) wishes. If no other physician or institution can be found, then the intervention may be withheld or withdrawn if this is in accordance with institutional policies and applicable state laws.

A patient's death caused by the termination of life support is not considered criminal because the patient's medical condition, rather than the termination of life support, is the cause of death. The removal of life support merely allows nature to take its course. When life support is terminated, the intent is to relieve suffering rather than to bring about the death of the patient. Furthermore, the intent of "comfort measures" is to ensure the relief of pain and suffering rather than to hasten the patient's death. Comfort measures (e.g., morphine) may indeed hasten death; this, however, is not the intention.

CHAPTER 47

The determination of brain death

Brain death is defined as the *permanent and irreversible loss of all brain function*. Most states in the United States consider brain death to be synonymous with the death of the patient. *The patient who is brain dead is dead.* The determination of brain death is a clinical diagnosis. The specific requirements for the determination of brain death vary from institution to institution and state to state. However, they all have a number of the following features in common:

- The recognition of the irreversibility of the brain insult requires that:

    The cause of brain death be established

    The insult be of a sufficient severity to account for the loss of the brain function

- A period of reasonable observation (and treatment) is required before the determination of brain death, to ensure irreversibility of brain damage.

    At least 6 hours if structural brain damage is present

    At least 12 hours if there is nonstructural brain damage

    At least 24 hours postcardiac arrest

    When drugs are implicated, the blood levels of these agents must be below therapeutic levels before the determination of brain death

    The patient's temperature must be > 34° C

    The patient must not be in shock

- Most institutions require that two physicians independently perform a clinical determination of brain death. The clinical findings must be clearly recorded in the patient's chart.
- Clinical determination of brain death:

  Absence of spontaneous movements, movements in response to pain, decerebrate or decorticate posturing

  Absent brainstem responses
  - Pupils fixed and nonresponsive to light
  - Absent corneal reflex
  - Absent cough and gag reflex
  - Absent "dolls eyes"

  Negative caloric test; no response (nystagmus) to the instillation of 50 ml of ice saline in each auditory canal

  Positive apnea test: preoxygenate patient with 100% oxygen. Obtain blood gas. Disconnect patient from the ventilator and insert an oxygen catheter down the endotracheal tube. Observe for spontaneous respiratory movements. After 10 minutes obtain a repeat blood gas (the $Paco_2$ increases by about 3 mm Hg/min). The patient is apneic if the $Paco_2 > 60$ mm Hg, and there are no respiratory movements. If the patient's baseline $Paco_2$ is low (due to hyperventilation) it is prudent to allow this to normalize before performing the apnea test.

- An number of ancillary tests can be performed to support the diagnosis of brain death. These tests are not required and in themselves are not sufficient to make the diagnosis of brain death. They are useful in the presence of toxic substances or sedative drugs

  Cerebral angiography: no blood flow on a four-vessel angiogram establishes the *irreversibility* of coma.

  Cerebral radionuclide studies: absent cerebral blood flow supports the diagnosis of brain death. Cerebral nuclide flow studies, however, are not as sensitive as four-vessel angiography for the determination of brain death.

Brainstem evoked potentials: the absence of brainstem evoked potential establishes the irreversibility of coma.

An isoelectric electroencephalogram (EEG), while compatible with brain death, may occur in patients with sedative overdose who subsequently "recover."

- In those states where brain dead patients are considered dead, the physician does not require the permission of the family or other individuals to remove a dead patient from mechanical ventilation or other life-support equipment. Organ donation should be considered in all brain dead patients. When the patient is being evaluated for organ donation, this must be discussed with the family and their consent obtained.

Management of the heartbeating, brain dead organ donor

Recent advances in surgical technology, organ preservation, immunosuppressive therapy, and life-support technology have allowed organ transplantation to play a major role in the treatment of patients with end-stage diseases that involve the thoracic and most of the abdominal viscera. Consequently, the demand for transplantable organs is increasing. Multiple organ retrieval from a single cadaver donor is an efficient means of procuring transplantable organs. In the United States alone, about 2 million people die each year, and of these about 12,000 to 27,000 individuals are suitable to donate organs. The donor pool necessary to meet current transplantation needs has been projected between 10,000 and 15,000 per year. Despite what seems to be an adequate donor pool, only 15% to 20% of potential donors become actual donors.

The refusal for organ donation by relatives, and unwillingness of health care providers to confront relatives with the diagnosis of brain death and requesting permission to procure organs are major reasons for loss of potential transplantable organs. Neglecting the general routine care of a potential donor before organ procurement will cause hemodynamic instability, infection, or unexpected cardiac arrest, leading to needless rejection of organs or tissues that otherwise would have been suitable for transplantation. Early donor recognition, rapid and accurate declaration of brain death, physiologic maintenance, and coordination with a local organ procurement agency are all important aspects of organ donor management.

After a potential donor is identified and consent is obtained or the patient has an organ donation card, the donor is evaluated for medical suitability, and a local organ procurement agency is contacted. It is important to assess the medical suitability of the donor and his organs. The various studies required for evaluation of the donor are listed in Table 48-1. However, all donors should be evaluated on an individual basis.

A few absolute contraindications apply to all potential organ donors, including HIV infection, other active viral infections (CMV, hepatitis A, hepatitis B, systemic herpes), history of intravenous drug use, malignancy (except primary CNS tumors), and concurrent sepsis. The organ-specific contraindications for organ donation are listed in Table 48-2.

Table 48-1 Workup of the organ donor

Donor organ	Test required
All donors	Height, weight, blood type, chem 7, ABG, CBC with platelets, PT, PTT, serology for HIV, CMV, EBV, toxoplasma, and hepatitis B; blood cultures if infection is suspected; lymph node biopsy for tissue typing may be required
Kidney	Urinalysis, BUN, creatinine, urine culture
Heart	ECG, ECHO, chest x-ray, CPK-MB, cardiology consultation, cardiac catheterization (in selected cases)
Lung	Chest x-ray, sputum Gram stain and culture
Liver	SGOT, SGPT, alk phosphatase, bilirubin
Pancreas	Amylase
Small bowel	Amylase

Table 48-2 Organ-specific donor criteria

Organ	Age	Laboratory parameters	Contraindications
Heart	Male <40 Female <45	Normal ECG, ECHO, CK-MB	Cardiomyopathy, valvular disease, congenital heart disease, chronic severe hypertension, severe chest trauma, open cardiac massage, prolonged (> 20 min) cardiac massage, high-dose dopamine (>10 μg/kg), abnormal ECG/ECHO or cardiac cath, CK-MB > 5%, PaO_2 <50 mm Hg for 4 hr
Kidney	>1 or <65	Urine output >0.5 ml/kg/hr, BUN <30 mg/dl, serum creatinine <1.5 mg/dl, creatinine clearance >70 ml/min	Pyelonephritis, chronic renal disease, severe hypertension, pyuria, bacteriuria, diabetes mellitus, hematuria, DIC, abnormal sediment
Lung	Male <40 Female <45	pO_2 >110 on FIO_2 <0.3, normal CXR, normal $AaDO_2$, normal airway pressures	Pulmonary edema, infection, penetrating thoracic trauma, smoking history, chronic lung disease, >24 hours of mechanical ventilation, positive sputum culture, pO_2 <60 mm Hg at FIO_2 >0.4 and PEEP >5 cm H_2O.

Liver	6 months to 55 years	Normal SGOT, SGPT, alk phosphatase, bilirubin,	Penetrating abdominal injury, chronic liver disease, alcohol abuse, hepatobiliary sepsis, RUQ surgery, dopamine >10 PT/PTT µg/kg/min, abnormal LFT, PT, PTT, Po_2 <50 for 4 hr
Pancreas	>2, <50	Normal amylase, lipase, glucose tolerance test	Pancreatitis, diabetes mellitus, gastric, duodenal or pancreatic surgery
Small bowel			Penetrating abdominal injury, elevated amylase
Heart valves	<60		Valvular heart disease, ECHO showing valvular deformity or dysfunction
Skin/bone			Local malignancies, local open injuries
Cornea	<90		Local injury, conjunctivitis

When the brainstem is dead, there is no possibility of recovery since both the capacity and the ability to breathe have been irreversibly lost. The process of dying has started, and although not every cell in the body has yet ceased to function, the subsequent death of the organism is inevitable. In adults, irreversible cardiac arrest usually occurs within 48 to 72 hours of brain death despite all efforts to maintain the donor's circulation.

During early brainstem herniation, peripheral vasoconstriction is seen due to increased sympathic activity. This is followed by loss of vascular tone, causing hypotension, venous pooling, and relative hypovolemia. Therapeutic dehydration (to decrease cerebral edema), incomplete fluid resuscitation, and diabetes insipidus may contribute to hypovolemia. Atrial and ventricular arrhythmias and various degrees of conduction block are not uncommon. They can be due to electrolyte imbalance, hypotension, myocardial ischemia, hypothermia, inotropic agents, myocardial contusion, and increased intracranial pressure. Despite all therapeutic efforts, all brain dead patients will have terminal arrhythmias resistant to therapy. Electrolyte abnormalities are frequent in organ donor patients. Diabetes insipidus is seen commonly after brain death as a result of partial or complete loss of production of ADH.

Brain dead patients are poikilothermic because they lack hypothalamic regulation of temperature. Hypothermia can lead to bradycardia, myocardial depression, arrhythmias, cold diuresis, coagulopathy, and left shift in the oxygen dissociation curve.

MANAGEMENT OF THE DONOR

The successful donation of perfusable organs requires continued maintenance of the patient's cardiac function, the correction of all electrolyte and metabolic derangements, and the use of artificial respiration until the moment of organ removal. The aims of management of organ donor are to maintain body temperature, prevent infection, and optimize the condition of transplantable organs.

- Establish a cause of death.
- Minimum monitoring includes, hourly measurements of temperature, pulse, blood pressure, and urine output. All patients will need a wide-bore intravenous cannula and Foley catheter. An arterial line is very helpful. Some may need CVP monitoring and a pulmonary artery catheter for fluid management.
- Check ABG; electrolytes, including calcium, magnesium, phosphate; CBC with platelets, PT, and PTT frequently.
- Hypotension is best managed by fluid resuscitation to obtain a systolic blood pressure of 90 to 100 mm Hg (Fig. 48-1).
- A urine output of at least 0.5 ml/kg/hr indicates adequate hemodynamics. If urine output is low despite adequate blood pressure, mannitol or furosemide may be used.
- Ventricular tachyarrhythmias, especially associated with hypothermia, respond best to bretylium tosylate.
- Bradyarrhythmias with hypotension are managed by dopamine infusion. This can be followed by an epinephrine infusion. Rarely, a transvenous pacemaker may be required. Atropine does help in this circumstance.
- Ventilation should achieve a normal pH, $Paco_2$, and O_2. CO_2 production falls after brain death, requiring a lower minute ventilation. Maintain adequate oxygenation ($Pao_2 > 70$ mm Hg) on the lowest possible Fio_2 (< 0.4 if lungs are to be used) and minimal PEEP (< 5 cm).
- Use strictly aseptic techniques when performing invasive procedures and endotracheal suction. Some centers use prophylactic antibiotics.
- A high urine output (> 4 ml/kg/hr) can be managed by replacing urinary losses with intravenous fluid

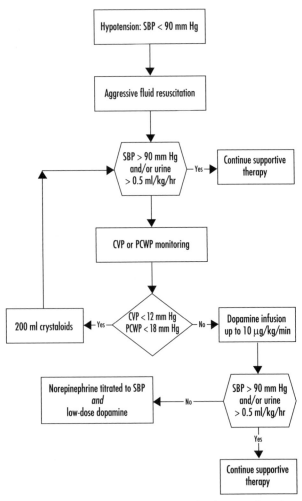

Fig. 48-1 Hypotension in the brain dead organ donor.

containing 0.45% saline with 30 mmol potassium phosphate/liter of fluid, on a volume-to-volume basis.

- Diabetes insipidus (urine output > 5 to 7 ml/kg/hr, urine specific gravity < 1005) is managed by synthetic vasopressin infusion (0.5 to 15 U/h) to decrease urine output to 2 to 3 ml/kg/hr.
- Control blood sugar (in the range of 140 to 240 mg/dl) with intravenous insulin to keep serum glucose in the range of 140 to 240 mg/dl.
- Some centers routinely use replacement doses of tri-iodothyronine and cortisol.
- Keep body temperature > 34° C (see Chapter 55).
- Keep hematocrit > 25% and platelet count > 30,000.

Multisystem
organ failure

With the widespread use of advanced organ support, patients rarely die from their presenting disease but rather die from its pathophysiologic consequences. Most patients who die in the ICU do so from multisystem organ failure (MSOF). See Table 49-1. Patients who have developed MSOF have an extraordinarily high mortality, and for many patients the support of MSOF does not improve survival but rather prolongs the dying process. The mortality rate is roughly proportionate to the number of organs that have failed and reaches 80% to 100% once three or more organs have failed (for over 7 days). Organ dysfunction is a spectrum varying from mild to severe.

Table 49-1 Classification of MSOF

System	Mild dysfunction	Moderate dysfunction	Severe dysfunction
Respiratory	$Pao_2/Fio_2 > 250$	Pao_2/Fio_2 150-250	$Pao_2/Fio_2 < 150$
Renal	Creatinine < 1.7 mg/dl	Creatinine 1.7-3.4 mg/dl	Creatinine > 3.4 mg/dl; need for dialysis
Hepatic	Bilirubin < 1.7 mg/dl	Bilirubin 1.7-4.7 mg/dl	Bilirubin > 4.7 mg/dl
GI tract	NG drainage < 300 ml/24 hr; diarrhea in response to enteral feeding	NG drainage 300-1000 ml/24 hr; visible blood drainage	NG drainage > 1000 ml/24 hr; upper GI bleed requiring transfusion; acalculous cholecystitis; pancreatitis
Cardiac	SVT	PCWP > 16 mm Hg; requires dobutamine/dopamine at < 10 μg/kg to maintain adequate cardiac output	Requires inotropic agents to maintain MAP > 80 mm Hg
CNS	GCS 13-14	GCS 10-12	GCS < 10
Hematology	Plt < 60,000	Plt 20,000-60,000 PT/PTT 1-1.5 × control	Plt < 20,000 PT/PTT > 1.5 × control
Metabolic	Insulin requirements < 1 U/hr	Insulin requirements 2-4 U/hr	Insulin requirements > 5 U/hr
Immunologic	Reduced delayed hypersensitivity	Cutaneous anergy	Cutaneous anergy + recurrent infection with ICU pathogens

CHAPTER 50

Sedation in the ICU

Almost all ICU patients require some form of sedation.

INDICATIONS

- To allay anxiety
- For patient comfort
- To permit mechanical ventilation
- To decrease oxygen requirements
- To protect patients from injuring themselves

RAMSEY SEDATION SCORE

- I. Anxious and agitated
- II. Cooperative, orientated, and tranquil
- III. Drowsy, responds to verbal commands
- IV. Asleep, responds briskly to light stimulation
- V. Asleep, sluggish response to stimulation
- VI. Asleep, no response to stimulation

TREATABLE CAUSES OF ANXIETY

- Uncontrolled pain
- Ventilator settings inappropriate—respiratory inco-ordination
- Drug or alcohol withdrawal syndrome

- Increased work of breathing, e.g., pneumothorax, kinked or blocked tube, pulmonary edema
- Loud ventilator alarms and monitors
- Poor communication with patient as regards diagnosis, therapy, etc.

THE SEDATION PLAN

- Aim to achieve Ramsey score II in nonintubated patients and III to V in intubated patients. Patients requiring greater ventilator support (i.e., high PEEP, high pressures, and high rate) require more sedation.
- Morphine and a benzodiazepine are the standard agents used for sedation in most ICU patients. Morphine should be used even in patients without obvious pain because it allays anxiety and potentiates the effects of benzodiazepines. Patients with pain will require larger doses of morphine.
- PRN orders should be *avoided* except when weaning from sedation. Sedation should be given at *regular timed intervals*, i.e., hourly or every two to four hours and titrated according to the patient's response. Administering regular timed dosages achieves much smoother sedation and reduces the total dosage of sedatives.
- Give supplemental sedation and an analgesic when performing painful procedures, e.g., dressing changes in a burn patient, line changes, cardioversion, etc.
- Use sedative agents very cautiously in patients with liver failure.
- Haloperidol, 2.5 to 20 mg IV every 15 minutes to every 6 hours is the drug of choice for acute delirium. This drug is also useful when patients become agitated and disorientated when being weaned from sedative drugs. Extrapyramidal effects and risk of neuroleptic malignant syndrome (NMS) are independent of dose.
- Propofol is a particularly useful sedative and anesthetic agent in the ICU. It is useful when rapid

emergence from sedation is required, in patients with hepatic and/or renal dysfunction, and in patients in whom deep sedation or anesthesia is required.

PHARMACOLOGIC AGENTS

Refer to Tables 50-1 and 50-2. The most cost-effective protocol is probably the combination of lorazepam (or diazepam) and morphine. Lorazepam (Ativan) has an intermediate duration of action, no active metabolites and may be given as intermittent boluses or as an infusion. Lorazepam should be used in patients with hepatic and/or renal failure when accumulation of active metabolites may become a problem. Diazepam (Valium) is insoluble in water, has a long half-life, and has active metabolites. Midazolam (Versed) has a short half-life, no active metabolites, and can be given as intermittent boluses or as a continuous infusion. Midazolam is particularly useful when short-term sedation is required. Tachyphylaxis occurs with all sedative agents, especially midazolam, resulting in a dosage escalation with an increasing length of sedation.

Propofol is a new IV anesthetic agent whose pharmacokinetic profile renders it suitable for prolonged sedation or anesthesia. A remarkable feature of the agent is the rapid and smooth recovery from anesthesia. Propofol is highly lipophilic, with very large volume of distribution and a short half-life. The beta-half-life is between 0.5 and 1 hours, with the liver being the most important site of elimination. After hours to days of infusion, one can expect a rapid decline in plasma concentration because of redistribution, with a smooth recovery. The pharmacokinetics are reportedly not significantly altered by hepatic cirrhosis or renal failure. Propofol is a potent vasodilator, and volume supplementation may be required to maintain the blood pressure. The drug is supplied as a 10% lipid solution, which significantly increases the patient's caloric intake (intralipid solutions should be stopped). Propofol has no analgesic properties, and therefore analgesics may be required.

Table 50-1 Benzodiazepine pharmacokinetics

Drug	Half-life (hr)	Dose equivalent (mg)	Active metabolites	Overall rate of elimination
Chlordiazepoxide	5-20	10	Desmethylchlordiazepoxide, demoxepam, desmethyldiazepam	Slow
Diazepam	30-60	5	Desmethyldiazepam	Slow
Lorazepam	10-20	1		Intermediate
Oxazepam	5-10	15		Interrapid
Midazolam	1-3	2		Rapid

Table 50-2 Dosages and duration of action of opiates

Agent	Usual initial IV dose	Duration of action
Morphine	3-5 mg	2-3 hr
Meperidine	20-25 mg	2-4 hr
Fentanyl	2-3 µg/kg	0.5-1 hr
Alfentanil	10-15 µg/kg	30 minutes

Propofol may be indicated in head injured patients in whom it is important to intermittently access the level of consciousness. In patients in whom neuromuscular paralysis is required, a propofol infusion titrated to achieve deep anesthesia (alone or in combination with a benzodiazepine) may allow avoidance of neuromuscular blocking agents. This alternative may prevent the postneuromuscular blockade "paralysis" syndrome. In patients who have been receiving long-term sedation with benzodiazepines and/or opiates, switching to a propofol infusion a day or two before weaning may allow a more rapid and smooth emergence.

Standard dosages of sedatives and hypnotics are as follows:

- Diazepam 2 to 10 mg, given 1 to 4 hourly
- Midazolam 2 to 10 mg, given 1 to 4 hourly
- Lorazepam 2 to 6 mg, given 1 to 4 hourly
- Morphine 2 to 10 mg, given 1 to 4 hourly
- Propofol infusion 0.5 to 3 mg/kg/hr

SEDATION PROTOCOL

Nonintubated patients (Ramsey II)

Dosage steps for Lorazepam IV are as follows:

Step 1: 1 mg q 12 hr
Step 2: 1 mg q 6 hr

Step 3: 1 mg q 4 hr
Step 4: 2 mg q 4 hr
Step 5: 4 mg q 4 hr

Assess level of sedation every 4 hours, if inadequate, give 1 mg bolus and then proceed to next dosage step. Reduce dosage step every 12 hours and reassess.

Intubated patients (Ramsey II-V)

Lorazepam and morphine infusion. Initial bolus: 2 mg lorazepam + 2 mg morphine, then infusion 2 mg/hr lorazepam + 2 mg/hr morphine.

Assess every 15 minutes until adequate level of sedation is achieved, and then every 6 hours. If inadequate, give 2 mg bolus of both lorazepam and morphine and then increase infusion rate by 1 mg/hr. Reduce infusion rate by 1 mg/ml every 12 hours, and then reassess.

ADJUNCTIVE SEDATION AND ANALGESIA FOR PERFORMING A PROCEDURE

A bolus of any of the aforementioned drugs may be used. Alternate agents include the following:

- Ketamine 0.5 to 1 mg/kg, provides excellent analgesia and anesthesia (in higher dose).
- Fentanyl 2 to 5 µg/kg, provides good analgesia.

FURTHER THOUGHTS

- Tachyphylaxis develops with all the sedative agents. The degree of sedation therefore needs to be frequently assessed and the dosage adjusted accordingly.
- In postoperative patients or patients with pain, transdermal fentanyl patches (which deliver 20/50/75 or 100 µg/hr) may provide excellent pain control.

- Low-dose opiate/bupivacaine epidural analgesia is particularly useful after abdominal procedures and in polytrauma patients.
- It is particularly difficult to assess the level of sedation in patients who are receiving neuromuscular blocking agents. Ensure that the patient is receiving high doses of sedative agents. Unexplained tachycardia, hypertension, and diaphoresis may be due to inadequate sedation.

CHAPTER 51

Neuromuscular blockade

The major indication for neuromuscular blockage in the ICU is to facilitate ventilation and reduce the risk of barotrauma in the following circumstances:

- When using high PEEP
- When peak airway pressures are high
- When using inverse-ratio ventilation or pressure-controlled inverse-ratio ventilation
- When using PEEP with low tidal volume ventilation
- Neuromuscular blockade may be used to facilitate crash intubations

Neuromuscular paralysis is sometimes used to reduce the work of breathing. This may favorably influence the pattern of oxygen utilization.

Neuromuscular blockade may cause significant morbidity and should only be used when absolutely indicated, and then only for the shortest possible period. Neuromuscular blockade should *never* be used for the treatment of anxiety or restlessness. All patients receiving neuromuscular blocking agents should be monitored using a nerve stimulator. For practical purposes the train of four (TOF) should be used to access the degree of neuromuscular blockade. The goal is to achieve one to two twitches (see p. 307).

PHARMACOLOGIC AGENTS

Pancuronium is probably the most cost-effective agent. In patients in whom the vagolytic and histamine releasing effects need to be avoided, e.g., in severe asthmatics or patients with a tachycardia, vecuronium or doxacurium can be used. In patients with hepatic or renal failure, atracurium (or doxacurium) should be used (pancuronium and vecuronium have active metabolites). Doxacurium and atracurium do not have a steroid structure and may be indicated in patients who are at risk of developing the "postparalysis paralytic" syndrome (i.e., patients receiving high-dose corticosteroids).

I.   *Pancuronium*: duration 120 to 150 minutes
    A. *Intubation*: 0.06 to 0.08 mg/kg
    B. *Maintenance*: 4 to 8 mg/hr
II. *Vecuronium*: duration 60 to 75 minutes
    A. *Intubation*: 0.07 to 0.1 mg/kg
    B. *Maintenance*: 4 to 10 mg/hr
III. *Atracurium*: duration 45 to 60 minutes
    A. *Intubation*: 0.4 to 0.5 mg/kg
    B. *Maintenance* 20 to 50 mg/hr
IV. *Doxacurium*: duration 30 to 160 minutes
    A. *Intubation*: 0.015 to 0.03 mg/kg
    B. *Maintenance* 0.005 to 0.03 mg/kg/hr
V.   *Succinylcholine (for intubation only)*: duration 5 to 15 minutes, 1 mg/kg. Beware of bradycardia with repeated doses.

Contraindications to the use of succinylcholine include the following:

- Renal failure
- Burns
- Severe trauma with muscle injury
- Severe sepsis
- Ocular injuries

TRAIN OF FOUR DOSAGE ADJUSTMENTS (TOF)

The train of four stimulus (four stimuli 0.5 seconds apart) is a convenient way of monitoring the degree of neuromuscular blockade and roughly correlates with the degree of neuromuscular junction receptor occupation.

- *Four twitches*:   0% to 70% receptors occupied
- *Three twitches*: 70% to 80% receptors occupied
- *Two twitches*:   80% to 90% receptors occupied
- *One twitch*:   > 95% receptors occupied
- *No twitches*:   100% receptors occupied

In principle, any superficially located peripheral motor nerve can be stimulated. The ulnar nerve is, however, the most popular site. The electrodes are best applied on the volar (palmar) side of the wrist. The distal electrode should be placed about 1 cm proximal to the point at which the proximal flexion crease of the wrist crosses the radial side of the tendon to the flexor carpi ulnaris muscle. The proximal electrode should be placed 2 to 3 cm proximal to the distal electrode. With this placement of electrodes, electrical stimulation normally elicits finger flexion and thumb adduction (Fig. 51-1).

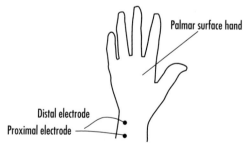

Fig. 51-1 Electrode placement for TOF stimulus.

Because different muscle groups have different sensitivities to neuromuscular blocking agents, results obtained for one muscle cannot be extrapolated automatically to other muscles. The diaphragm is the most resistant of all muscles to neuromuscular blockade. In general, the diaphragm requires 1.4 to 2 times as much muscle relaxant as the adductor pollicis muscle for an identical degree of blockade. From a practical point of view, two or three twitches (of train of four) of the adductor pollicis muscle will result in sufficient diaphragmatic paralysis to prevent the patient from coughing, hiccoughing, and breathing during mechanical ventilation.

Before paralysis, the supramaximal stimulation (SMS) must be determined. The SMS is defined as the level at which additional stimulation current does not increase the twitch response. It is important to note that each nerve may have a different SMS, and inadequate stimulation may lead the clinician to overestimate the degree of neuromuscular blockade present. The SMS is usually in the range of 20 to 60 mA.

Starting at 10 mA, increase the TOF current by 10 mA until four equal responses are obtained. Continue to increase the current until the intensity of the response does not increase any further. When this occurs, the prior setting will be the SMS for that nerve. Once the patient is paralyzed, the TOF is then performed using the SMS.

The TOF test should be performed hourly until the goal is achieved (two or three twitches) and then 6 hourly. The rate of the infusion may be adjusted as follows:

- *No twitches*: stop infusion, restart when two twitches are present. Restart infusion rate at:
     80% if it takes 1 hour for two twitches
     75% if it takes 2 hours for two twitches
     50% if it takes 3 hours for two twitches
     25% if it takes 4 hours for two twitches
- *One twitch*: reduce to 80% of present infusion rate
- *Two twitches*: maintain present infusion rate

- *Three twitches*: maintain present infusion rate; reload with 25% of loading dose and increase infusion rate by 25% if patient coughs, hiccoughs, or breathes over the ventilator
- *Four twitches*: reload with 50% of loading dose; increase infusion rate by 25%

Enteral and parenteral nutrition

"There is no disease process that benefits from starvation." All critically ill patients should receive early nutritional support.

THE METABOLIC RESPONSE TO SEPSIS AND TISSUE INJURY

- As part of the acute stress response, the levels of the following hormones and cytokines are increased:
    Catecholamines
    Cortisol
    Growth hormone
    Glucagon/insulin ratio
    Aldosterone
    Alpha-TNF
    IL-1 and IL-6
- The following metabolic changes are a consequence of this altered hormonal milieu:
    Impaired glucose oxidation $\Rightarrow$ hyperglycemia

    Muscle proteolysis and albumin catabolism with release of amino acids
        Gluconeogenic amino acids $\Rightarrow$ hepatic gluconeogenesis $\Rightarrow$ hyperglycemia

    Synthesis of acute phase reactants, cytokines, IgG, complement

Hypoalbuminemia
Peripheral lipolysis

Hyperglycemia and increased FFA $\Rightarrow$ hepatic lipogenesis

Insulin resistance with an impairment of glucose utilization is a common metabolic consequence of sepsis and tissue injury. The reduced glucose uptake provokes greater mobilization of fat reserves (lipolysis) and fat oxidation. It therefore appears that fat is the preferred fuel in this situation. Exogenous insulin does not correct this metabolic derangement, and hyperglycemia should be treated by reducing the glucose load. Recent experimental clinical data suggest that an infusion of somatostatin and insulin may normalize the aberrant glucose kinetics in patients with sepsis and multiorgan dysfunction.

NUTRITIONAL ASSESSMENT

- *Integrity and function of the bowel*
- Premorbid conditions, e.g., cardiac failure, alcoholism, AIDS, geriatric malnutrition
- Severity of acute insult
- Length of time starved
- Biochemical indicators, e.g., albumin, prealbumin, transferrin

NUTRITIONAL REQUIREMENTS

- Can be *measured* by indirect calorimetry and nitrogen balance or *estimated* using a number of formulas
- Studies have demonstrated that in about 50% of patients the Harris-Benedict equation may overestimate energy requirements by about 1000 kcal/day
- There are no data to suggest that accurately measuring nutritional requirements improves outcome

- The complications of overfeeding include hepatic steatosis with hepatic dysfunction, elevated BUN and blood sugar, and excessive CO_2 production
- The recommended average daily requirements are as follows:

  Nonprotein calories ± 25 to 30 kcal/kg/day

  CHO: MAX 4 mg/kg/day (± 1600 kcal)

  The body cannot utilize (oxidize) more than 4 mg/kg/day of glucose. Excess glucose administration will result in hyperglycemia and lipogenesis. Lipids should be 4 to 12 kcal/kg/day

  Protein: 1.5 to 2 g/kg/day

  Water-soluble vitamins, fat-soluble vitamins, and trace elements

Resting energy expenditure calculated by indirect calorimetry (Weir equation)

REE (kcal/day) = $[V_{O_2} (3.94) + V_{CO_2} (1.11)] \times 1440$

One can see from this equation the major impact that oxygen consumption has on energy expenditure.

Basal energy expenditure calculated by the Harris-Benedict equation (kcal/day)

Men: $66 + (13.7 \times \text{weight in kg}) + (5 \times \text{length in cm}) - (6.8 \times \text{age in years})$

Women: $655 + (9.6 \times \text{weight in kg}) + (1.8 \times \text{length in cm}) - (4.7 \times \text{age in years})$

Estimated energy expenditure from the BEE and disease state the following:

- Postoperative × 5%
- Peritonitis × 5% to 10%
- Long bone fracture × 15% to 30%
- Severe infection, multiple trauma × 30% to 55%
- Multiple trauma and mechanical ventilation × 50% to 70%

- Burns: 10% BSA × 25%
                  20% BSA × 50%
                  40% BSA × 80%
                  50% BSA × 100%
                  70% BSA × 120%

ROUTE OF FEEDING (Table 52-1)

The route of administration is an important consideration when optimizing nutritional support for critically ill patients. Studies in both animals and humans have provided strong evidence that enteral nutrition, but not parenteral nutrition, is a valuable adjunct to therapy in postoperative and critical care patients. A metaanalysis of eight prospective randomized studies (in trauma patients) has demonstrated that early enteral nutrition is associated with a lower infection rate and shorter length of ICU stay compared with TPN. Consistent with these studies are the results of the multicenter Veteran Affairs Total Parenteral Nutrition Cooperative Study, which indicated that perioperative TPN is associated with increased postoperative infectious complications.

A strong body of evidence supports the conclusion that early enteral nutrition (in trauma, burn, postoperative, and other critically ill patients) reduces the extent of bacterial translocation and improves the hormonal, metabolic, and immunologic derangements that occur with acute injury. Clinically this translates into a reduced incidence of infectious complications and decreased length of hospital stay.

All attempts should be made to feed the bowel. TPN should be considered a "dangerous" and suboptimal alternative route of feeding critically ill patients. Unless the patient has an ischemic bowel or loss of bowel continuity, the gut should be fed.

Inaudible bowel sounds and the absence of stool and flatus does not mean that the bowel is nonfunctional and cannot accept feeding. This thinking is outmoded and has been disproven. Surgeons have shown that early jejunal feeding can be suc-

Table 52-1 Advantages of enteral feeding over TPN

	Enteral	TPN
Bowel	Stimulates release of enteric hormones and increases splanchnic blood flow; maintains mucosal integrity	Mucosal atrophy, translocation of bacteria
Metabolic	Metabolic complications are less frequent	Hyperchloremic acidosis, hyperglycemia, hypophosphatemia, hypercapnia
Catheter-related complications	NIL	Increased incidence of catheter sepsis, complications of catheter insertion
Anabolism	Anabolic	Very difficult to achieve positive nitrogen balance in critically ill patients receiving TPN; TPN, however, limits catabolic loss of protein
Immunologic	Immunomodulating properties: "immunoenhancing" enteral formulas available	*May* have deleterious effect on immune system
Cost and ease	Simple and economical	More complex and expensive

cessful even when begun in the recovery room after major abdominal surgery. Even when one has to resort to TPN, small volumes (20 ml) of enteral feed should be given to the patient to limit the degree of gut mucosal atrophy.

Enteral feeding: if the bowel works, use it (Table 52-2)

Critically ill patients often have gastroparesis. An ileus affects the stomach first, the colon next, and the small bowel last (recovery occurs in the reverse order). Therefore before initiating enteral feeding, the choice between gastric and small bowel access should be made. If the gastric residual is less than 150 ml and the patient is not at high risk for aspiration, gastric feeding should be attempted. If the residual is larger or the patient is refluxing, the risk of aspiration is greater, and small bowel feedings are a better choice. If the patient will require surgery, an open abdomen provides the opportunity for placement of small bowel tubes.

During the first 24 hours following admission to the ICU, enteral feedings that provide 50% of the patient's nutritional needs should be commenced. This should then be advanced to 100% of the patient's calculated needs by 72 hours. If gastric residuals become large (>150 ml) and/or should the patient reflux, the stomach should be emptied and the feeding then restarted at one half the volume. *Cisapride*, a relatively new and unique prokinetic agent, improves gastric emptying in critically ill patients and may prove useful in patients who have large residuals and/or tolerate tube feeding poorly. Cisapride can be added to the enteral feedings at a dose of 10 mg every 6 hours. Should the residual remain high and/or the patient tolerates tube feeding poorly, postpyloric access should then be obtained.

Postpyloric intubation may be achieved by a number of methods. A jejunal feeding tube can be placed endoscopically or under radiographic screening. A number of double-lumen feeding tubes are available that allow postpyloric feeding and simultaneous gastric aspiration. It is possible

Table 52-2 Constituents of common enteral formulas (1000 ml)

Product	Calories	CHO (g)	Protein (g)	Fat (g)	Na (mEq)	K (mEq)	Osmolarity (mosm/kg)
Ensure	1060	140	36	36	32	30	470
Ensure Plus	1500	197	54	53	50	60	690
Ensure Plus NH	1500	197	62	49	52	47	650
Osmolite	1060	143	37	38	24	26	300
Osmolite HN	1060	139	43	36	40	40	300
Impact	1000	130	56 (L-arginine)	28	48	36	375
Jevity	1060	150	44	36	40	40	310
Hep Aid II	1180	170	40 (branch chain AA)	40	15	< 5	560
AminoAid	2000	370	20 (essential AA)	50	0	0	850
Vivonex	1000	190	45	10	25	30	650

to place a postpyloric tube at the bedside by the using the following method (some practice is required):

- A feeding tube with a wire stylet is required
- Place the patient on his or her right side (NB)
- Remove the nasogastric tube (NB)
- Lubricate the tube and insert through the nares until the stomach is reached ($\pm$ 40 cm). Remove the stylet and inject air into the stomach to confirm placement in the stomach
- Make a 30- to 45-degree bend in the last 3 to 4 cm of the stylet. Lubricate the stylet and then reinsert it into the feeding tube
- Using a "corkscrew" action, advance the feeding tube. Increased resistance is felt when the pylorus is entered (withdraw tube and readvance until the pylorus is "felt"). Advance the tube as far as possible. Remove the stylet and do the following:

    Inject air to confirm postpyloric placement by injecting air (less tympanic sound and heard lower down)

    or

    Aspirate through the tube and test pH with litmus paper
- Confirm position radiographically
- Reinsert nasogastric tube

In some patients transpyloric intubation may be difficult. However, spontaneous transpyloric passage of the tube may occur. This may be aided by nursing the patient with the right side down and giving a prokinetic agent. A recent study has suggested that a nonweighted tube is more likely to pass through the pylorus than a weighted tube.

A small amount of methylene blue should be added to the formula, making regurgitation easier to detect. Enteral feeding should always be given as a continuous infusion, rather than as intermittent boluses. A continuous infusion has the following advantages, compared with bolus feeding:

- Less diarrhea
- Less gastric discomfort

- Less hyperglycemia
- Lower risk of aspiration

Recent data suggest that specific nutrients directly modulate the host's inflammatory and immune response. Specifically, enteral nutrition supplemented with arginine, RNA, and omega-3-fatty acids have been shown to significantly improve the immunologic and metabolic derangements characteristic of critical illness and to improve clinical outcomes (septic complications, organ failure, and length of stay) in select groups of patients. Although these formulations are more expensive, they are probably cost-effective in the following clinical situations:

- Patients requiring mechanical ventilation for longer than 48 to 72 hours
- Patients with multisystem organ dysfunction or failure
- Patients with serious bacterial and/or fungal infections; e.g., abdominal sepsis, nosocomial pneumonia
- Polytrauma
- Burns (requiring admission to an ICU)
- Following major gastrointestinal surgery

PARENTERAL NUTRITION

- Data suggest that a standard TPN formulation is adequate for 80% to 90% of patients. Adjustments in the rate of infusion and volume will meet most patients needs:

    400 g CHO (dextrose; 1360 kcal) + 70 g protein in 1.5 to 2 liters

    250 ml of 20% fat solution (500 kcal)
- *Starting TPN*: start slowly—50% of goal first day, 75% of goal second day, 100% of goal third to fourth day.
- *Stopping TPN*: TPN should not be suddenly stopped (may cause profound hypoglycemia). Gradually reduce the infusion rate as enteral feeding is started.
- *TPN and the liver*: most complications occur within a month of starting TPN and include both biochemical and histologic abnormalities.

Biochemical

Increase in transaminases, usually 1 to 2 weeks after starting TPN

Transaminases usually normalize without stopping or changing TPN

Bilirubin and alkaline phosphatase may also increase

Histologic

Steatosis

Lipidosis

Cholestasis

Steatohepatitis

Etiology: caused by excessive CHO infusions and ? essential fatty acid deficiency

Management

Provide 20% to 50% of nonprotein calories as fat

Use medium chain triglycerides

Stop copper and manganese supplementation

Administer small amounts of lipids and protein enterally

NUTRITION IN LIVER FAILURE

- It is a common (and serious) error to limit protein intake in patients with liver failure. A high-protein diet has been shown to result in improvement of encephalopathy and hepatic function
- *Use* 60 to 80 g/day standard amino acid diet
- The use of aromatic or branch chain amino acids is of unproven value

NUTRITION IN RENAL FAILURE

- *Acute renal failure*: 1 g/kg of balanced amino acid diet and optimal nonprotein calories.
- *Chronic renal failure*: ketoanalogues may be useful in patients with decreased protein intake for more than 1 week

- Patients receiving TPN and continuous renal replacement therapy; amino acid intake should be increased 30%

NUTRITION IN PANCREATITIS

- IV lipids are safe if TGs are monitored
  TG should be < 400 mg/dl during infusion
  TG should be < 200 mg/dl after infusion (1 hour)
- Preliminary data suggest that duodenal-jejunal feeding with a low-fat elemental diet does not stimulate pancreatic secretions and may be safe in pancreatitis

COMMON FEEDING ERRORS IN THE ICU

- Not using a functioning bowel
- Waiting too long before initiating feeding; the amount and type of "feed" is less important than the delay in initiating nutritional therapy
- Stopping nutrition abruptly, e.g., when the patient is going to the operating room or when the patient is to be extubated. In this circumstance, supplement with 10% dextrose water IV to prevent *hypoglycemia*
- Hyperglycemia indicates glucose intolerance; reduce the glucose intake. *Do not* increase the insulin infusion (maintain glucose between 140 and 220 mg/dl).

THE REFEEDING SYNDROME

Protein-calorie malnutrition has been shown to exist in up to 50% of hospitalized patients. Feeding malnourished patients, particularly after a period of starvation may result in severe metabolic disturbances, most notably hypophosphatemia. Hypophosphatemia developing after initiating parenteral or enteral nutrition has been termed the *refeeding syndrome*. In addition to hypophosphatemia, changes in potassium, magnesium, and glucose metabolism occur during refeeding. Although classically described in cachectic patients after prolonged starvation, this syndrome has been reported to occur commonly in poorly nourished ICU patients who have been starved for as short as 48 hours.

In the starved individual the catabolism of fat and muscle leads to loss of lean muscle mass, water, and minerals. Despite a reduction in total body phosphate, the serum concentration generally remains in the normal range because of adjustments in the renal excretion. With conversion to carbohydrate as the major energy source during refeeding, insulin release is stimulated. Carbohydrate repletion and insulin release together enhance the uptake of glucose, phosphorus water, and other components into the cell. The combination of total body phosphorus depletions and increased influx of phosphorus during refeeding leads to severe extracellular hypophosphatemia. Low serum phosphorus levels lead to depletion of high-energy phosphate bonds and ATP, altering cellular metabolism. Hypophosphatemia as an isolated metabolic abnormality has been found to impair organ function and may result in severe sequelae (see Chapter 25).

The commercially available tube feed preparations contain between 50 and 60 mg/dl (the recommended daily allowance). However, in patients with high metabolic demands and in phosphorus-depleted patients, these formulas may not meet the requirements necessary to accommodate the massive transcellular shifts and possible whole-body depletion of phosphorus found in these patients.

In patients with poor baseline nutrition, refeeding should commence slowly and gradually. Serum levels of potassium, phosphate, and magnesium need to be determined before refeeding and monitored daily during the first week of refeeding.

CHAPTER 53

Assessment of
tissue oxygenation

GENERAL PRINCIPLES

Tissue hypoxia is common in critically ill patients and is likely a major contributing factor leading to organ failure. The expedient detection and correction of tissue hypoxia may limit organ dysfunction, shorten ICU stay, and improve the outcome of patients treated in the intensive care unit. In studying oxygen utilization in critically ill patients, the following factors are important:

- Measurements of systemic oxygen delivery (Do_2) and consumption (Vo_2) provide no information as to the adequacy of tissue oxygenation. A patient may have a high oxygen delivery and yet have an oxygen debt; similarly a patient may have a subnormal oxygen delivery in the absence of tissue hypoxemia. Systemic oxygen delivery and consumption must therefore be interpreted in conjunction with indexes of tissue oxygenation.
- Changes in regional blood flow and oxygen utilization cannot be predicted from changes in systemic oxygen utilization. In septic patients, systemic oxygen delivery is increased, yet the nutrient blood flow to the liver, kidneys, and intestines may be markedly reduced. In cardiorespiratory disease, when systemic oxygen delivery is reduced, the liver, kidneys, and intestines become ischemic earlier, and to a greater

degree than predicted from changes in systemic oxygen transport.

- It has been widely suggested that increasing oxygen delivery to above 600 ml/min/M^2 may improve the outcome of critically ill patients. Optimization of the preoperative hemodynamic profile has been shown to improve the outcome of high-risk surgical patients. When applied to the general ICU population, this therapeutic maneuver is unproven and potentially dangerous. A number of studies have shown that increasing oxygen delivery to predetermined levels improves outcome; however, other studies have provided contradictory results.

- Gastrointestinal ischemia is an early manifestation of impaired tissue perfusion. This may result in disruption of the intestinal mucosa allowing for the translocation of bacteria and bacterial products into the circulation. It has been suggested that this process may trigger a cascade of events that produces further tissue ischemia resulting in multisystem organ failure (MSOF).

- Blood lactate levels are determined by the balance of whole-body production and liver metabolism. Normal blood lactate levels may occur in the presence of organ ischemia. Hepatic function and hepatic blood flow significantly influence blood lactate levels. It has been demonstrated that for a similar degree of oxygen debt, the serum lactate level is significantly higher in patients with cardiogenic as opposed to septic shock. This is a consequence of the greater hepatic blood flow in septic as opposed to cardiogenic shock.

- A consequence of cellular oxygen deprivation is a severe intracellular metabolic acidosis. This can occur in the absence of lactate production. Its cause is not completely understood; however, it is believed to result from the unreversed hydrolysis of ATP (i.e., $ATP \rightarrow ADP + Pi + H^+$). Extracellular tissue acidosis results from intracellular acidosis. It follows that determining the cellular (or interstitial fluid) redox state or pH may be particularly useful for detecting early organ-specific tissue hypoxia.

- Data suggest that the earlier an oxygen debt is detected and corrected the greater the likelihood that the intervention will improve outcome. Once tissue acidosis has developed or organ failure manifests clinically, it is likely that the cycle of progressive organ dysfunction has been entered. Under such circumstances it is unlikely that an intervention that increases oxygen delivery will significantly impact patient outcome.

- As tissue oxygen delivery decreases, oxygen extraction increases. Analysis of PVO_2 may provide an indication of the adequacy of tissue oxygenation. A PVO_2 of less than 35 mm Hg is usually indicative of tissue hypoxia while a PVO_2 of less than 30 mm Hg is a sign of severe tissue oxygen deprivation. However, PVO_2 analysis in septic patients can be misleading; because of an abnormality of oxygen utilization or extraction, the PVO_2 may be normal (or high) in septic patients despite profound tissue hypoxia.

- Gastric tonometry is a simple and minimally invasive tool that allows for the indirect determination of gastric intramucosal pH (pHi). The pHi has been shown to correlate well with splanchnic oxygen delivery and the adequacy of tissue oxygenation. The measurement of pHi in critically ill patients may allow for the early detection of tissue ischemia and inadequate oxygen delivery.

GASTRIC TONOMETRY

Tonometry is simply a method used to equilibrate gas tension between two compartments. Either gas (e.g., helium) or fluid (e.g., normal saline or gastric fluid) can be used as the solvent for equilibration of the gas in question (i.e., carbon dioxide). Tonometry can be performed in any hollow viscus. Although tonometry has been performed in the large bowel and bladder, most experience has been gained with gastric tonometry. A nasogastric tonometer is a standard nasogastric tube with a silicone balloon at its distal end.

Gastric intramucosal pH can be computed by substituting the gastric intramural P_{CO_2} and gastric intramural HCO_3^- into the Henderson-Hasselbalch equation. However, neither intramural P_{CO_2} or intramural HCO_3^- can be measured directly. Nevertheless, intramural HCO_3^- can be estimated by measuring arterial HCO_3^-, if it is assumed that gastric intramural and arterial HCO_3^- are similar. This premise holds true except in situations where there is "no flow" to the stomach (i.e., celiac artery occlusion). Furthermore, studies have shown the gastric mucosa to be highly permeable to intramural CO_2 and that the intramural CO_2 rapidly equilibrates with the CO_2 dissolved in gastric fluid. Therefore intramural P_{CO_2} can be determined by measuring the P_{CO_2} of gastric juice. Rather than aspirating gastric juice and determining its P_{CO_2} directly, intraluminal P_{CO_2} can be inferred by measuring the P_{CO_2} of saline contained within a silicone balloon positioned within the stomach (a gastric tonometer). Since silicone is very permeable to CO_2, the P_{CO_2} of the intraluminal fluid and P_{CO_2} of the saline in the balloon tend to equilibrate rapidly in a predictable time-dependent manner.

Measurement of the pHi

Gastric mucosal pH as measured by tonometry has been validated by direct measurement using microelectrodes. Furthermore, experimental data have demonstrated the pHi to be linearly related to the intramucosal pH in the small and large intestine and to the hepatic venous lactate concentration. The pHi therefore indirectly reflects the adequacy of splanchnic aerobic metabolism.

Before insertion, the tonometer port is flushed with normal saline to eliminate air. The tonometer is then inserted into the stomach either through the nose or mouth. The position of the tube must be confirmed radiologically.

The balloon of the tonometer is filled with normal saline and allowed to equilibrate (ideally for 90 minutes) with the intragastric Pco_2. Once equilibrated, the balloon is aspirated, and the Pco_2 of the fluid is determined using a standard blood gas analyzer. The Pco_2 is corrected for the equilibration time using a correction factor. The pHi is then calculated by substituting the Pco_2 and arterial HCO_3^- concentration into the Henderson-Hasselbalch equation. The normal pHi is 7.39 ± 0.03.

MEASUREMENT OF TISSUE OXYGENATION

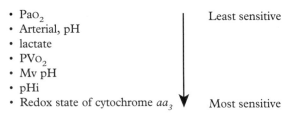

- Pao_2 — Least sensitive
- Arterial, pH
- lactate
- PVo_2
- Mv pH
- pHi
- Redox state of cytochrome aa_3 — Most sensitive

As can be seen from Fig. 53-1, there is a steep oxygen diffusion gradient from the lungs to the arterial blood, to

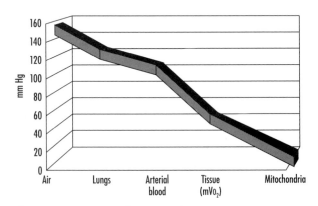

Fig. 53-1 Oxygen diffusion gradient.

the tissues, and to the mitochondrion. Oxygen is the final electron receptor in the respiratory chain. A partial pressure of oxygen only 1 to 2 torr is required in the mitochondrion to maintain aerobic metabolism. The redox state of cytochrome aa_3, as measured by near infrared spectroscopy (NIH), is the best tool available to measure intramitochondrial P_{O_2}. However, NIH is not widely available for clinical use. The PV_{O_2} and pHi are indirect estimates of the adequacy of tissue oxygenation. However, the PV_{O_2} is unreliable in patients with sepsis. As cellular and tissue acidosis are early signs of tissue hypoxia, monitoring pHi may be a useful tool for detecting early tissue hypoxia.

CHAPTER 54

Blood component therapy and coagulopathies

INDICATIONS

- Red cells

  Chronic anemia (Hb < 8.5) with evidence of cardiac decompensation

  Acute anemia (Hb < 7.5) with cardiac compromise or inadequate tissue oxygenation

  Acute GI tract bleed with Hb < 10
- Platelets

  Chronic thrombocytopenia (< 5000) and patient bleeding

  Acute or chronic thrombocytopenia (< 20,000) and patient on chemotherapy

  Acute or chronic thrombocytopenia (< 50,000) and patient bleeding

  Acute or chronic thrombocytopenia (< 100,000) and operative bleeding

  Contraindicated in TTP

- Fresh frozen plasma

  Replacement of clotting factors when PT and/or PTT 1.5 × control or greater and patient bleeding or facing hemostatic challenge

  Treatment of thrombocytopenic purpura (TTP)
  Treatment of ATIII deficiency

- Cryoprecipitate
   Fibrinogen < 100 mg/dl and patient bleeding
   Hemophilia A or von Willebrand disease

NOTE: Fresh frozen plasma contains all the stable and labile plasma constituents. One unit of FFP contains approximately 400 mg of fibrinogen and 1 unit clotting activity per milliliter.

Cryoprecipitate is prepared from a cold insoluble precipitate of plasma. It contains high levels of factor VIII (both procoagulant activity and von Willebrand factor) and fibrinogen. The other clotting factors are not present in sufficient amounts to be of therapeutic value.

DOSING GUIDELINES

Refer to Table 54-1.

THE "OPTIMAL HEMATOCRIT": HOW MUCH IS ENOUGH?

Traditional wisdom in anesthesia has always held that patients should have a hemoglobin concentration > 10 g/dl (HCT > 30) before the administration of anesthesia for surgery. Similarly it has been taught that the hemoglobin of critically ill patients should be kept above 10 g/dl. The value of 10 g/dl is based on the theoretical premise that the arterial oxygen content should be greater than the oxygen extraction of tissue with the highest extraction, which for clinical purposes is the myocardium whose oxygen extraction is 12 ml/dl. This postulate was erroneously supported by a number of poorly designed clinical experiments. This simplistic view overlooks the physiologic adjustments seen in acute stress that serves to maintain adequate oxygen delivery and ignores the myriad of deleterious effects associated with blood transfusion.

There is a lack of reliable data to define the ideal hemoglobin concentration in critically ill patients. A

Table 54-1 Dosing guidelines for using blood components

Blood component	Dose	Recommended infusion times
Fresh frozen plasma	Two units (400-600 ml)	1 hr
Platelets	Use whatever dose is necessary to increase platelet count above 50,000; six units are usually sufficient; or one unit of platelets per 10 kg	30 min
Cryoprecipitate	Desired increase in g/L = (0.2 × number bags)/ plasma volume in L; or use one bag/5 kg	IV push or 100 U/10 min
Packed red blood cells	One unit increases hemoglobin by 1.0-1.5 g/dl	2-3 hr

number of authors have failed to demonstrate an improvement in global and organ-specific oxygenation when critically ill patients with a hemoglobin of less than 10 g/dl are transfused. Indeed, recent data suggest that the number of units of transfused blood may be an independent predictor of MSOF and death.

The National Blood Resource Education Program and the NIH guidelines state that "adequate oxygen carrying capacity can be met by a *hemoglobin of 7 g/dl (HCT of approximately 21%)* or less when the intravascular volume is adequate for perfusion." They, however, do add the caveat that the hemoglobin concentration should be maintained above 7.5 g/dl in patients with poor cardiorespiratory function.

Risks and adverse affects associated with red cell transfusion include the following:

Infectious

Cytomegalovirus	Common
Non-A, non-B hepatitis	1:100 (before hepatitis C screening)
Hepatitis B	1:100 to 1:200
HIV	1:40,000 to 1:1,000,000
Bacterial sepsis	Rare

Immunologic

Fever, chills, urticaria	1:50 to 1:100
Acute hemolytic t/f reaction	1:12,000
Delayed hemolytic t/f reaction	1:1000
Fatal hemolytic t/f reaction	1:100,000
Anaphylaxis (lgA or lgG)	1:150,000
Graft vs host reaction	Unknown
T/f related acute lung injury	1:5000
Pulmonary leukoagglutination syndrome	
Passive transfer of leukocyte agglutinating or cytotoxic antibodies	

Febrile nonhemolytic reaction of 1:100 to 1:200
   Recipient antibodies to donor WBCs

Immunoparesis
   Impaired B- and T-cell function

Other

An acute (transitory) neutrophilic leucocytosis

Increased blood viscosity

Microcapillary occlusion caused by transfusion of poorly deformable RBCs

Hyperkalemia

Metabolic alkalosis

Hypothermia

THE EFFECTS OF MASSIVE TRANSFUSION

- A massive transfusion is defined as the administration of blood in excess of one blood volume within 24 hours (approximately 10 U blood).
- *Dilutional coagulopathy*: prophylactic platelet transfusions and FFP are not recommended. The coagulopathy should be treated on a individual basis, dependent on the patient's clinical condition, the platelet count, and the PT and PTT.
- *Citrate toxicity and hypocalcemia*: citrate toxicity is uncommon except in patients with underlying liver disease (citrate is metabolized to lactate and bicarbonate by the liver) and patients receiving in excess of 40 U blood. Calcium should only be given to patients with a low ionized serum calcium (< 1 mmol/L).
- *Electrolyte and acid-base*: hyperkalemia and alkalosis may develop after a massive transfusion.

ALTERNATIVES TO TRANSFUSION OF BLOOD COMPONENTS

- Red cell substitutes
    Perfluorocarbon emulsions
        Do not have a significant effect on oxygen transport. Oxygen carrying capacity is highly dependent on the partial pressure of oxygen:
            50 ml/100 ml at Pao_2 of 600
            0.3 ml/100 ml at Pao_2 of 100 mm Hg
        Have significant toxicity
    Other experimental solutions have not been clinically tested
        Polymerized hemoglobin solutions
        Liposome embedded hemoglobin
        Stroma-free hemoglobin
- Recombinant erythropoietin (EPO). EPO shows promise as an adjunctive agent in the treatment of anemia accompanying both acute and chronic illness.

The agent is very expensive, and its role has yet to be determined.
- Desmopressin (DDAVP) increases plasma factor VIII:c and promotes release of von Willebrand factor from endothelial stores. DDAVP increases platelet function in patients with uremia, cirrhosis, and aspirin ingestion.

COAGULATION DISORDERS AND DISSEMINATED INTRAVASCULAR COAGULATION (DIC)

Coagulation disorders are commonly encountered in the ICU. Many conditions including sepsis, malignancy, trauma, vasculitic disorders, and obstetric accidents may give rise to a coagulopathy. In addition patients may have medical conditions that predispose them to developing a coagulopathy, e.g., patients with liver disease, renal failure, lupus, or leukemia. Sepsis, however, is the most common factor leading to a coagulopathy.

The clinical and laboratory findings will depend on the precipitating factors. Patients usually have features of a consumptive coagulopathy and clinical features of both bleeding and thrombosis. End organ damage is usually due to microvascular thrombosis. A microangiopathic hemolytic anemia may occur.

- Laboratory features
  Peripheral blood smear will show fragmented red blood cells and thrombocytopenia with large platelets

  Prolonged PT and PTT
  Thrombocytopenia
  Decreased levels of fibrinogen
  Decreased levels of antithrombin III

  Increased levels of fibrin split products and D-dimer
- Clinical features associated with bleeding
  Bleeding from venipuncture sites, mucous membranes, hematuria, GI bleeding, intracerebral bleeding

Petechia, purpura, and subcutaneous hematomas
- Clinical features of end organ damage caused by thrombosis
    Acute lung injury syndrome
    Proteinuria and renal insufficiency
    Budd-Chiari syndrome, hepatocellular dysfunction
    Mental state changes and neurologic deficits
- Management
    The most important aspect of the management of DIC involves the treatment of the precipitating factors

    In patients with bleeding complications, clotting factors should be replaced (per guidelines above)

The use of heparin in patients with DIC is controversial. Heparin is indicated in patients with acute promyelocytic leukemia and perhaps patients with DIC associated with solid tumors. Low-dose heparin may be useful in patients with DIC who have thrombotic complications. Antithrombin III concentrates may also be useful.

CAUSES OF THROMBOCYTOPENIA IN THE ICU

- Bacterial sepsis is perhaps the most common cause of thrombocytopenic in the ICU. Thrombocytopenia is often an early sign of sepsis. Many factors lead to platelet activation and consumption.
- Dilutional as a result of blood and fluid replacement
- Consumptive coagulopathy (DIC) caused by sepsis, liver failure, HELP syndrome, abruptio placentae
- Microangiopathic hemolytic anemia, i.e., thrombotic thrombocytopenic purpura (TTP), hemolytic uremic syndrome (HUS)
- Immune thrombocytopenias
    Idiopathic (ITP)
    Alloantibodies
    Collagen vascular diseases
    Malignancy

Viral

Drug-induced (quinidine)

- Myelosuppressive chemotherapeutic agents
- Heparin-associated thrombocytopenia syndrome (HATS)
- Infiltrative marrow diseases, neoplastic, TB
- Drugs are commonly implicated in the cause of thrombocytopenia. Almost any drug can cause a thrombocytopenia. The commonly implicated drugs include the following:

Antimicrobials

Chloramphenicol

Amphotericin

Tetracyclines

Sulfonamides

Penicillins

Cephalosporins

Anticonvulsants

Phenytoin (Dilantin)

Carbamazepine

Diuretics

Furosemide

Thiazides

Ethacrynic acid

Others

Alcohol

Phenylbutazone

Aspirin

Gold salts

Colchicine

Chlorpromazine

Chlordiazepoxide

Cimetidine and other H_2-blockers

HEPARIN-ASSOCIATED THROMBOCYTOPENIA

There are three different syndromes of heparin induced thrombocytopenia:

- *Acute reversible thrombocytopenia*: this is seen immediately after an intravenous bolus injection of heparin. It is thought to be due to reversible clumping, trapping, and sequestration of platelets caused by a direct effect of heparin. The acute reversible thrombocytopenia is mild and associated with no deleterious effects.
- Mild thrombocytopenia, with platelet counts between 100,000 and 150,000, developing 2 to 4 days after initiation of heparin therapy. The platelet count typically returns to normal within 1 to 5 days.
- A delayed and persistent thrombocytopenia associated with heparin resistance, DIC, and thromboembolism. The onset of the thrombocytopenia occurs between day 6 and 14, is usually severe, and platelet counts recover rapidly once the heparin is discontinued. The syndrome is independent of the dose of heparin, and has been described with heparin bonded catheters. This syndrome is associated with heparin-dependent platelet antibodies. Arterial and venous thrombosis and skin necrosis have been described in this syndrome, often called the *white clot syndrome*.

HEPARIN RESISTANCE

Refer to Chapter 12.

CHAPTER 55

Accidental hypothermia

Accidental hypothermia is defined as the unintentional decline in the core body temperature below 35° C. The compensatory physiologic responses to hypothermia are limited and fail below a temperature of 35° C. Usually there is a history of obvious environmental exposure. However, subtle presentations are common in the elderly. Hypothermia is usually graded as mild, moderate, or severe (Table 55-1).

CONDITIONS ASSOCIATED WITH HYPOTHERMIA

- Advanced age
- Hypothyroidism
- Hypoadrenalism
- Environmental exposure
- Chronic debilitating diseases, such as cardiac failure, renal failure, or strokes
- An acute cerebrovascular accident, especially in the elderly, with immobility and poor thermoregulatory mechanisms
- Drugs
  Ethanol
  Phenothiazines
  Tricyclic antidepressants
  Barbiturates

Table 55-1 Physiologic changes associated with various degrees of hypothermia

Severity	Body temperature	Nervous	Cardiac	Other
Mild	32.2-35° C 90-95° F	Amnesia, dysarthria, apathy, confusion, shivering, ataxia	Tachycardia, then progressive bradycardia, vasoconstriction, cold	Tachypnea, then hypoventilation, bronchospasm, cold diuresis
Moderate	28-32.1° C 82.4-89.9° F	Decreased LOC, dilated pupils, hallucinations, hyporeflexia, rigidity	Decreased pulse and cardiac output, arrhythmias, J waves, cardiac conduction slows with prolonged PR, QRS and QT intervals and ventricular irritability increases	Hypoventilation, decreased urine, coagulopathy (despite normal levels of clotting factors), lactic acidosis, depressed hepatic function
Severe	< 28° C < 82.4° F	Coma, loss of ocular reflexes, no movement, areflexia	Progressive fall in pulse and BP, arrhythmias, asystole	Pulmonary edema, apnea, oliguria, rhabdomyolysis, hemoconcentration, hyperglycemia, increased transaminases, hyperamylasemia

MANAGEMENT

- Monitoring

    The core temperature should be continuously monitored (rectal, bladder, and/or esophageal)

    Bladder catheterization to monitor urine output
    Continuous electrocardiographic monitoring

    Frequent check of electrolytes: hyperkalemia is not uncommon; hypothermia masks the typical ECG changes of hyperkalemia.
    Acid-base evaluation:

    Arterial blood gas analyzers warm the blood to $37°$ C and report the values directly so that arterial blood gas values do not need to be corrected for the patient's lower body temperature. The use of uncorrected values permits reference to standard nomograms. The use of uncorrected arterial blood gas values as a guide to resuscitation is called the *ectothermic strategy*.

    When blood cools, the pH increases, and the $Paco_2$ falls. The pH of neutrality is 7.5, and the $Paco_2$ is 30 mm Hg at a temperature of $30°$ C

- Rewarming (Fig. 55-1)

    Active external rewarming

    Involves direct exposure of the patient's skin to any exogenous heat source

    Includes immersion, radiant heat, forced air, and heating blankets

    Complications include thermal injury and peripheral vasodilation with core temperature afterdrop
    Active core rewarming

    Heated humidified air: inhalation of air humidified and heated (via a mask or endotracheal tube) to a temperature of $40°$ C will raise the core body temperature by about $1°$ to $2°$ C per hour.

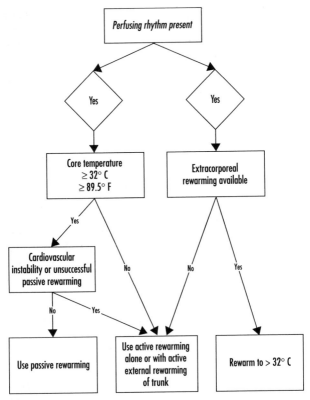

Fig. 55-1 Hypothermia.

Administration of intravenous fluids heated by countercurrent heat exchangers up to 42° C

Peritoneal lavage with 10 to 20 ml/kg of dialysate heated to 40° C at a rate of 6 L/hr will raise core temperature by about 2° C to 4° C/hr

Gastric, colonic, and bladder irrigations should be avoided because they may lead to unwanted complications

Mediastinal irrigation via chest tubes has been recommended by some investigators. This invasive procedure may be associated with many complications.

Extracorporeal venovenous warming has been shown to be a very efficient and reasonably simple method of rewarming.

Extracorporeal rewarming using the standard cardiopulmonary bypass circuit. Femoral catheterization with flow rates of 2 to 3 L/min will raise the core temperature 1° C to 2° C every three to five minutes. Although cardiopulmonary bypass is the most rapid means of increasing the core body temperature, this procedure is impractical for most patients because it requires specialized personnel and equipment; arterial and venous cutdowns are usually required; and it is usually restricted to the operating room.

- Supportive medical therapy

  Because of cold-induced diuresis, decreased fluid intake and third-space loss, patients usually have a decreased intravascular volume and require volume replacement (sometimes massive)

  Ringer's lactate should not be given to severely hypothermic patients because the liver cannot convert lactate to bicarbonate, making the metabolic acidosis worse

  Airway protective reflexes are commonly lost in the hypothermic patient, necessitating intubation and mechanical ventilation

  Insertion of a pulmonary artery catheter may incite ventricular ectopy and ventricular fibrillation and should be avoided. In hemodynamically unstable patients and/or patients with underlying cardiac disease pulmonary artery catheterization should be delayed until the patient's core temperature is above 32° C

Rhabdomyolysis should always be excluded and aggressively managed if present (see Chapter 29)

Vasoactive agents may precipitate severe arrhythmias. Low doses may be used in severely hypotensive patients who have failed to respond to fluids.

Bretylium is the antiarrhythmic agent of choice

Pharmacologic agents are usually ineffective below a temperature of 30° C. Drugs such as atropine are therefore ineffective

Myxedema and hypoadrenocorticism should be excluded. Patients should be treated with corticosteroids if there is a clinical suspicion of adrenal insufficiency. However, the empiric administration of parenteral levothyroxine to euthyroid patients with hypothermia is hazardous. An urgent serum TSH level should almost always be performed and intravenous levothyroxine given in myxedematous patients.

Exclude infection. Many of the signs and symptoms of infection, including fever and leukocytosis are obscured by hypothermia

Hypothermic patients have a coagulopathy with an increased tendency to bleed (inactivation of coagulation enzymes and platelet destruction by cold). Some patients, however, may develop DIC.

Nasogastric intubation to prevent vomiting and aspiration

CHAPTER 56

Burns

BURN MANAGEMENT

- *Estimate extent of burn*
    "Rule of nines" for rapid approximation of % BSA
    The area of patient's palm ~ 1% BSA
- *Estimation of depth of burn*
    Partial thickness
        Pink or mottled red
        Wet appearance
        Covered with vesicles or bullae
        Painful
    Full thickness
        Charred
        Dry appearance
        Thrombosed superficial veins
        Insensate
- *Indications for admission to ICU or burn center*
    Adults > 25% BSA
    Children > 20% BSA
    Full thickness burns > 10% BSA
    Burns of face, hands, feet, eyes, ears, or perineum
    High-voltage electric injury
    Inhalation injury or associated trauma

    Medical conditions that increase the patient's medical risk
- *Fluid resuscitation*

IV hydration mandatory for all burns > 15% BSA
Ringer's lactate 2 to 4 ml/kg per % BSA burn in
first 24 hours, of which 50% is given in the first
8 hours

Colloid solution 0.3 to 0.5 ml/kg per % BSA burn
second 24 hours

Intravascular volume should be assessed continu-
ously (see Chapter 18) by monitoring BP, pulse,
urine output, as well as CVP, and in some instances
PCWP
- Other therapeutic interventions
  Tetanus toxoid
  Analgesia
  Wound care

  Bronchoscopic evaluation of airways with inhalational injuries or face burns

  Escharotomy to prevent compartment syndrome
  High-protein enteral feeding
  Stress ulcer prophylaxis

CARBON MONOXIDE POISONING
AND SMOKE INHALATION

All patients suffering from smoke inhalation should be
evaluated for thermal injuries to the upper airways, inhala-
tional smoke injuries, CO poisoning, and cyanide poisoning.
- Thermal injury to upper airways
  Result in laryngeal edema and laryngospasm
  Diagnosed by direct laryngoscopy

  Treatment: observation, humidification, airway toilet,
  and ? elective intubation
- Smoke inhalation
  Damages type 2 pneumocytes
  Results in bronchospasm, bronchitis, broncho-
  pneumonia, ARDS

  Diagnosed by presence of sooty sputum and
  bronchoscopic examination

- Cyanide poisoning

  Thermal decomposition of various nitrogen-containing material (such as wool, silk, polyurethane) produces hydrogen cyanide

  Delay in escape from fire results in prolonged exposure to toxic gasses

  Blood cyanide concentration is significantly elevated in fire victims, the level correlating well with the carbon monoxide level

  Increased lactate levels serve as a marker for cyanide toxicity

  Treatment:
  - 100% oxygen

    Hydroxocobalamin (combines with CN to form cyanocobalamin—vitamin B_{12})

    Nitrite therapy is potentially hazardous in cases of combined poisoning with carbon monoxide and cyanide

- CO poisoning

  Common sources
  - Engine exhaust
  - Fires
  - Furnaces and heating systems
  - Propane powered machinery
  - Indoor skating rinks
  - Indoor barbecue

  CO binds to hemoglobin and cellular enzyme systems (cytochrome a_3 and P450) interfering with oxygen transport and tissue oxygen utilization

  Symptoms
  - Acute (Table 56-1)

    "Chronic poisoning": asthenia, headaches, abnormal behavior, impaired memory or vision, occupational difficulty

Acute CO poisoning is associated with a syndrome of "delayed neurologic sequelae." Autopsies have shown degeneration and necrosis of the globus pallidum in these cases. Symptoms include a parkinsonian-like syndrome, intellectual deterioration, memory impairment, and personality changes

Treatment

100% oxygen by face mask

Treatment of associated injuries and cyanide poisoning

The role of hyperbaric chambers is controversial. This therapeutic modality may reduce the incidence of delayed neurologic sequelae. Hyperbaric oxygen therapy should be considered in patients who are stable enough to be transported to a hyperbaric facility and undergo this therapy. Placing an unstable patient in a hyperbaric chamber is associated with significant morbidity and mortality.

Table 56-1 Correlation of symptoms with carboxyhemoglobin concentration in carbon monoxide poisoning

Symptoms	Percent saturation of hemoglobin with CO
No symptoms	0-10
Tightness across forehead and headache	11-20
Headache and throbbing temples	21-30
Severe headache with nausea and vomiting and dimmed vision	31-40
Syncope, tachypnea, tachycardia	41-50
Coma and convulsions	51-60
Cardiovascular collapse, respiratory failure	> 60

Preoperative evaluation of the surgical patient

The goal of the preoperative medical assessment of the surgical patient is to assess the risk-benefit ratio of surgery, to identify factors increasing perioperative complications, and to optimize the patients health before surgery. This assessment done in advance is cost-efficient because it reduces delays on the day of surgery, allows optimization of the patients condition, and reduces the perioperative morbidity and mortality. This assessment is best performed well in advance of surgery and not on the evening before surgery.

The risks associated with surgery are dependent on the patient's age, physiologic health, underlying medical conditions, as well as the nature of surgery which is to be performed. The most accurate method of risk stratification is a thorough history and physical examination, followed by appropriate tests related to the patient's clinical condition (Table 57-1).

PREOPERATIVE INVESTIGATIONS

- *Chest x-ray*: data would suggest that the risks associated with chest radiographs probably exceed their possible benefit if the patient is *asymptomatic* and younger than 75 years of age. Chest x-rays should be performed in patients with a history of cardiorespiratory disease.
- *ECGs*: all patients above the age of 40 years should have a screening ECG.

Table 57-1 Mortality risk (%) for elective surgery determined by various degree of coexisting disease

Preoperative condition	Minor impairment	Major impairment	Poor function
Impairment of general health	1.4	4.9	21.5
Ischemic heart disease	1.6	4.3	40.1
Chronic lower respiratory infection	0.9	3.7	19.8
Cardiac failure	4.1	7.5	20.8
Obesity	0.3	2.2	14.6
Impaired renal function	2.8	4.4	22.5
Diabetes	1.6	5.8	14.9

- *CBC*: all female patients, all male patients over age of 65, and all symptomatic patients should have a screening CBC.
- *Blood chemistries*: no blood chemistries are warranted in patients less than 65 years of age, except for patients with a history of hepatic, renal, cardiovascular, or endocrinological disorders. BUN and glucose are recommended for patients greater than 65 and 75 years of age respectively.
- *Coagulation tests*: PTT and PT are only recommended in patients with a history of a coagulation disorder.
- *Pulmonary function testing*: data suggest that preoperative lung function testing in selected patients provides important information regarding the potential for postoperative respiratory morbidity. Patients with the following signs and symptoms should have preoperative PFTs:

  Patients with any evidence of COPD

  Smokers with a history of persistent cough

Patients with a history of wheezing or dyspnea on exertion

Patients with chest wall and spinal deformities

Morbidly obese patients

Patients undergoing thoracic surgery

Patients over the age of 70 years

Patients undergoing upper abdominal surgery

Pulmonary function parameters that predict increased postoperative risk:

$Pa_{CO_2} > 45$ mm Hg

$FEV1 < 2$ L

$FVC < 50\%$ predicted

$MVV < 50\%$ predicted

General anesthesia should be avoided in patients with a $FEV1 < 1$ L and/or $FVC < 30\%$ predicted, since it is almost certain that these patients will have a prolonged and complicated postoperative course with a high perioperative mortality.

In patients undergoing pulmonary resection, the postoperative FEV1 can be determined by using ventilation-perfusion scanning to determine the amount of functioning lung to be removed. A predicted postoperative FEV1 of greater than 1 L is an acceptable indicator of success after pulmonary resection.

Postoperative FEV1 = preoperative FEV1 ×
percent function of remaining lung from V/Q scan

PREOPERATIVE ASSESSMENT OF THE CARDIAC PATIENT

Cardiovascular complications account for approximately 50% of all deaths in patients undergoing noncardiac surgery, and more than 90% of these occur in patients with coronary heart disease. Cardiac patients with a high risk of postoperative infarction and cardiac death can be identified by a careful history and physical examination, followed by ECG, chest x-ray, and, where needed, Holter monitoring, echocardiograms, and either an exercise or dipyridamole-thallium stress test. In patients with ischemic heart disease it is necessary to evaluate both left ventricular function and coronary reserve (Table 57-2).

As is evident from Fig. 57-1, most perioperative infarctions occur between the first and fourth postoperative day. Up to 60% of perioperative infarctions occur silently and carry a high mortality. It therefore follows that patients at risk of suffering a postoperative infarction should be closely monitored for at least 4 days after surgery.

Cardiac contraindications to elective noncardiac surgery

- Myocardial infarction < 6 months (< 3 months if immediate surgery necessary)
- Overt heart failure
- Severe aortic stenosis
- Unstable angina
- Mobitz type II, complete AV block, sick sinus syndrome

Table 57-2 Approximate incidence of perioperative myocardial infarction in patients with previous myocardial infarction

Time from AMI (months)	1960	1975	1985
0-3	55%	37%	6%
4-6		16%	3%
7-12	25%	5%	
12-24	22%	5%	< 2%
> 24	6%	5%	

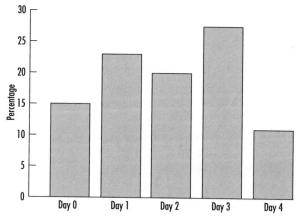

Fig. 57-1 When MIs occur after surgery.

Factors that decrease the risk of elective noncardiac surgery

- Coronary artery bypass surgery
- Successful angioplasty with EF > 40%
- Negative exercise stress test
- Absence of silent ischemia or frequent multiform ventricular premature contractions on Holter monitoring
- Ejection fraction > 40%

Patients undergoing vascular surgery are at the highest risk for cardiac events. Patients undergoing abdominal aortic aneurysm repair pose a considerable risk because of the magnitude of the myocardial stress imposed during aortic cross-clamping. Furthermore, most patients with abdominal aortic aneurysms will have coronary artery disease, and many will have hypertension and/or renovascular disease. Preoperative assessment of these patients includes either treadmill exercise testing, or bicycle ergometry, or dipyridamole-thallium imaging, or dobutamine stress echocardiography with cardiac catheterization in those patients with a positive test.

PREOPERATIVE OPTIMIZATION

Heart failure

Optimization of medial therapy with the combination of ACE inhibitor, digoxin, and titrated use of furosemide reduces the operative risks. Patients with an enlarged left ventricle, S_3 gallop, 2 or more episodes of cardiac failure, and or ejection fraction less than 40% require preoperative and postoperative hemodynamic monitoring.

Ischemic heart disease

- Preoperative, perioperative, and postoperative use of beta-blockade, if not contraindicated
- Nitrates commencing 6 hours preoperatively and for 48 to 96 hours postoperative
- Adequate control of heart failure for a few months before surgery
- Low-dose aspirin
- Perioperative hemodynamic monitoring

High-risk operative patients

Preoperative pulmonary artery catheterization with optimization of the hemodynamic profile, together with postoperative care in an ICU has been demonstrated to reduce perioperative morbidity in vascular surgery and other high-risk surgical patients.

Hemoglobin

A hemoglobin above 8 g/dl is adequate for nonblood loss surgery. In patients in whom significant bleeding is expected, the hemoglobin should be above 10 g/dl (HCT 30). Autologous blood should be considered in patients who are expected to require intraoperative or postoperative transfusions. Patients with a HCT above 55 should be venesected before surgery.

Pulmonary function

Smokers should stop smoking at least 4 weeks before surgery. Patients with reversible airways disease (bronchospasm) should receive maximal bronchodilator treatment. A course of antibiotics may be indicated in patients with chronic bronchitis. Elderly patients and patients with chronic pulmonary disease should receive preoperative instructions regarding breathing exercises and incentive spirometry.

Diabetics

Blood sugars should be well controlled before surgery. The following perioperative insulin regimens are recommended:

Night control regimen

- *Day before surgery*: the patient should be given nothing by mouth after midnight; a glass of orange juice should be at the bedside for emergency use.
- *6 AM on day of surgery*: institute intravenous fluids using a 5% dextrose solution infused at a rate of 125 ml/hr/70 kg of body weight.
- *After institution of intravenous infusion*: give one-half the usual morning insulin dose (and the usual type of insulin) subcutaneously.
- Continue 5% dextrose throughout the operation, giving at least 125 ml/hr/70 kg of body weight.
- In the recovery room, monitor blood glucose concentrations, and treat on a sliding scale.

Tight control regimen

- On the evening before the operation, determine preprandial blood glucose.
- Start an intravenous infusion of 5% dextrose water at a rate of 50 ml/hr/70 kg of body weight.
- Piggyback to the dextrose an infusion of regular insulin (50 units in 250 ml of 0.9% sodium chloride)

and an infusion pump. Before attaching this piggy-back line to the dextrose infusion, flush the line with 60 ml of infusion mixture and discard the flushing solution. This approach saturates the insulin-binding sites of the tubing.

- Set the infusion rate, using the following equation: insulin (U/hr) = plasma glucose (mg/dl)/150.
- Repeat measurements of blood glucose every 4 hours as needed, and adjust insulin appropriately to obtain blood glucose levels of 100 to 200 mg/dl.
- *The day of surgery*: dextrose and insulin infusion as outlined above.

Adrenal suppression

Patients who have received 5 mg (or equivalent) or more of methylprednisolone for 2 weeks or more should receive "stress" replacement doses of corticosteroids.

- 100 mg of hydrocortisone the evening before surgery
- 100 mg of hydrocortisone 1 hour before surgery
- 100 mg of hydrocortisone during surgery
- 100 mg of hydrocortisone every 6 hours for 24 hours
- For uncomplicated cases, decrease the dose by 50% per day until the regular maintenance dose is achieved

CHAPTER 58

Central venous catheterization

THE SUBCLAVIAN VEIN

- *Advantages*: consistent identifiable landmarks; easier, long-term catheter maintenance; relatively high patient comfort.
- *Disadvantages*: pneumothorax (1% to 2%) and subclavian artery puncture (1%). Subclavian catheterization is a relative contraindication in patients with a coagulopathy and/or pulmonary compromise (dependent on the expertise of the operator).
- *Anatomy*: it is continuation of axillary vein, beginning at the outer border of the first rib, extending 3 to 4 cm along the undersurface of the clavicle and joining the ipsilateral internal jugular vein behind the sternoclavicular joint (Fig. 58-1).
- *Position (most important)*: the patient is placed supine with arms at the side and head turned to opposite side, 15- to 30-degree Trendelenburg position, with a small bedroll placed between the shoulder blades.
- *Infraclavicular approach*: identify the clavicle, the suprasternal notch, and the acromium-clavicular junction. The operator's position is next to the patient's ipsilateral shoulder. Feel along the inferior border of the clavicle moving from medial to lateral, until you feel a "give" in the tissue resistance. This point is approximately at the junction between the medial and middle thirds of the clavicle and at the

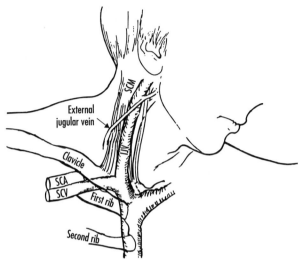

Fig. 58-1 Major veins of the neck. *SCM*, Sternocleido-mastoid; *IJV*, internal jugular vein; *SCA*, subclavian artery; *SCV*, subclavian vein.

point of the first "S bend" in the clavicle. The skin and subcutaneous tissue should now be infiltrated with 1% lidocaine. The thumb of the left hand is now placed "in" the suprasternal notch, to serve as a landmark. A 2¾ inch, 14-gauge needle is mounted on a syringe and directed cephalad from the "point" until the tip abuts under the clavicle. With the needle hugging the inferior edge of the clavicle, the needle is now advanced toward the suprasternal notch (the thumb of your left hand). The needle is advanced until the subclavian vein is entered.

- *Supraclavicular approach*: the operator's position is at the head end of the patient, on the ipsilateral side. Identify the clavicular insertion of the sternocleido-mastoid muscle and the sternoclavicular joint. The site of skin puncture is just above the clavicle and lateral to the insertion of the clavicular head of the sternocleidomastoid muscle. Advance the needle toward the contralateral nipple just under the clavicle. The needle is inserted at a 10- to 15-degree angle from the coronal plane, and it should enter the jugulo-subclavian bulb at 1 to 4 cm.

INTERNAL JUGULAR VEIN

- *Advantages*: minimal risk for pneumothorax, preferred in patients with hyperinflation and those receiving mechanical ventilation
- *Disadvantages*: carotid artery puncture (2% to 10%); not recommended if platelet count < 50,000 and elevated PT or PTT
- *Anatomy*: it emerges from the base of the skull through the jugular foramen and courses posterolateral to the internal carotid artery in the carotid sheath and runs beneath the sternocleidomastoid muscle (Fig. 58-1).
- *Position* is supine with 15-degree Trendelenburg and the patient's head turned gently to the opposite side
- *Central approach*: the skin is punctured at the apex of the triangle formed by the two muscle bellies of sternocleidomastoid muscle and the clavicle, at a 30- to 45-degree angle with the frontal plane and directed at the nipple on the same side
- *Anterior approach (recommended)*: the needle is inserted at the midpoint of the sternocleidomastoid muscle, approximately 5 to 6 cm from both the angle of the mandible and the sternal notch (four finger breadths), while feeling the carotid artery pulsation with the other hand and keeping the needle lateral to the pulsations. Introduce the needle at a 30- to 45-degree angle with the frontal plane, and direct caudally, parallel to the carotid artery toward the nipple on the same side. If the initial attempt is unsuccessful, direct the needle more laterally.
- *Posterior approach*: the needle is introduced 1 cm dorsal to the point where the external jugular vein crosses

the sternocleidomastoid muscle and is directed caudally and ventrally toward the suprasternal notch at an angle of 45 degrees with the sagittal plane, with a 15-degree upward angulation.

- *Finder needle*: a 22-gauge "finder" needle may be used to localize the internal jugular vein and avoid inadvertent internal carotid artery puncture with the wider bore needle. When venipuncture has occurred with the finder needle, either withdraw the finder needle and introduce a large-bore needle in same plane, or leave it in place and introduce a larger needle directly above it.

EXTERNAL JUGULAR VEIN (*NOT* RECOMMENDED)

- *Advantages*: no risk of pneumothorax and bleeding can be controlled; can be used in patients with severe coagulopathy
- *Disadvantages*: difficulty in advancing the catheter into the internal jugular vein
- *Anatomy*: it forms at the angle of the mandible behind the ear, and it runs obliquely across the sternocleidomastoid muscle and joins the subclavian vein behind the medial third of the clavicle (Fig. 58-1).
- *Position*: supine with arms to the side and head gently turned to the opposite side. May need to place patient in 15-degree Trendelenburg position to distend the vein.
- *Approach*: the venipuncture is done with 16-gauge needle using the left index finger and thumb to distend and anchor the vein. The guidewire is threaded up to 20 cm. Passage of the guidewire may be facilitated by abduction of the ipsilateral arm and anteroposterior pressure on the clavicle. Avoid using excessive force to advance the guidewire and catheter.

FEMORAL VEIN (RECOMMENDED)

- *Advantages*: *safe*, easily accessible, convenient during CPR, don't need Trendelenburg. The risk of infection is not increased when compared to other sites. Safe to perform in patients with a coagulopathy.
- *Disadvantages*: may be associated with an increased risk of thromboembolism. Limits flexion of leg at hip.
- *Anatomy*: it is continuation of popliteal vein and becomes external iliac vein at inguinal ligament. It lies medial to femoral nerve and femoral artery in the femoral sheath at the inguinal ligament.
- *Technique*: clean and shave the area. The patient is placed supine with the leg extended and slightly abducted at hip. Palpate for the femoral arterial pulsation; the site of puncture is 1 to 1.5 cm medial to the femoral arterial pulsation below the inguinal ligament. In a patient with no palpable femoral pulse, it is 1 to 1.5 cm medial to the junction of medial third and lateral two thirds of a line joining the anterior superior iliac spine and pubic tubercle. A 14-gauge needle is placed at the site of puncture and advanced at a 45- to 60-degree angle to the frontal plane with the tip pointed cephalad. After obtaining return of venous blood, the syringe and needle are depressed to skin level and free aspiration of blood reconfirmed.

CATHETER INSERTION TECHNIQUE

- Strict aseptic precautions are essential. Proper attire including gown, sterile gloves, mask, and cap is necessary. The site is prepared with povidone-iodine solution scrubs.
- *Seldinger technique*: when the vein is entered, the syringe is detached from the needle, and the guidewire with flexible J tip is inserted through the needle (sometimes the J tip does not advance easily; in this

situation attempt using the straight end of the guidewire). The needle is then removed over the guidewire.
The guidewire is then used to direct the catheter into
the vein. It is essential to never lose control (and sight)
of the guidewire. The catheter system is passed over
the guidewire until it rests in the lumen of the vessel.
The guidewire is then removed and the catheter is left
in place and secured with sutures. The tip of the
catheter (except for femoral insertions) should lie
at the junction of the superior vena cava and right
atrium. Central venous catheters advanced into the
right atrium have been associated with right atrial perforation. Generally, an internal jugular catheter should
be advanced to the 10 cm mark and a subclavian
catheter to the 15 cm mark (at the skin).

- *Postinsertion chest film*: chest films (preferably upright
  in expiration) are recommended after all attempts at
  central venous catheterization to determine the position of the catheter tip, and to exclude a pneumothorax, hemothorax, and/or cardiac tamponade.
- When venous access cannot be obtained by blind
  insertion of the needle, Doppler ultrasonography with
  visualization of the vein may be helpful. Alternatively,
  a venous cutdown may be required (saphenous,
  cephalic, basilic, external jugular, or femoral vein).

ANTECUBITAL VEINS (*NOT* RECOMMENDED)

- Commonly known as the *PICC line* (peripherally
  inserted central catheter)
- *Advantages*: no risk of pneumothorax, minimal
  bleeding
- *Disadvantages*: infection, thrombosis, low success
  rate, time consuming
- *Anatomy*: long catheters (up to 24 inches long) can
  be placed into the basilic or cephalic vein in the ante-
  cubital fossa and then threaded into the thorax. The

basilic vein lies along the medial aspect of the ante-
cubital fossa, and then ascends on the medial aspect
of the arm to form the axillary vein. The cephalic vein
lies along the lateral aspect of the fossa and ascends
along the lateral border of the biceps muscle

- *Position*: arm straight, patient need not be supine
- *Approach*: the basilic vein is preferred because of a
less variable course; right side preferred because of
shorter distance to superior vena cava. The vein is
distended with a tourniquet and entered under direct
vision. The catheter is advanced up to the manubrio-
sternal junction from the venipuncture site

COMPLICATIONS OF CENTRAL VENOUS ACCESS

- Venous air embolism: entry of air into the central
venous system through the catheter can be fatal. It is
best prevented by positioning the patient in a 15-degree
Trendelenburg position during catheter insertion. It
will manifest as tachypnea, wheezing, hypotension, and
"mill wheel" murmur over precordium. The patient
should be immediately turned onto her left side, in the
Trendelenburg position, and air aspirated after advancing the catheter into the right ventricle
- *Venous thrombosis*: common, usually of little clinical
significance, mural thrombi in 10% to 20% of cases
but clinically significant in only up to 3% of patients
- Local infection and catheter-associated bloodstream
infection.
- Pneumothorax and/or hemothorax occurs as a result of
injury to pleura and underlying lung; small pneumothorax can be observed, but medium to large pneumothoraces will require chest tube insertion
- *Arterial puncture*: if it occurs, apply sufficient pressure
for at least 10 minutes. Arterial puncture may be confirmed by pulsatile flow and high hydrostatic pressure
- Catheter tip migration and perforation of free wall of
cardiac chamber

- *Vascular erosions*: uncommon, typically occur 1 to 7 days after catheter insertion, cause sudden dyspnea with new pleural effusion or hydromediastinum on chest radiograph, more common with left sided catheter placement
- *Occlusion of catheter*: is common and best treated by replacement of catheter
- *Retained catheter fragment*: catheter tips may get sheared off by traction on beveled tip of inserting needle or by fracture of catheter caused by improper fixation and excessive movement
- *Inadvertent venous catheter placement*: into internal jugular vein or opposite subclavian vein from subclavian vein approach is not uncommon

TECHNIQUES FOR VASCULAR ACCESS WHEN VENOUS ENTRY IS IMPOSSIBLE

- Route for vascular access depends on the urgency and agent to be administered
- *Intraosseous*: intraosseous needle into proximal tibia can be used for fluids and drug administration
- *Arterial access*: intraarterial infusion of fluids, packed cells, and certain medications is possible into radial, brachial, femoral, iliac, and aorta
- *Endobronchial*: naloxone, epinephrine, atropine, diazepam, and lidocaine can be given endobronchially in volumes of 5 to 10 ml
- *Corpora cavernosa*: large volume of fluid can be infused via the corpora cavernosa for short term; avoid using any drugs via this route

The obstetric patient

PREECLAMPSIA AND ECLAMPSIA

- Diagnosis of pregnancy-induced hypertension (pre-eclampsia)
  Blood pressure:
  Systolic ≥ 140 mm Hg
  Diastolic ≥ 90 mm Hg

  Or increase in systolic blood pressure of 30 mm Hg or diastolic of 15 mm Hg from baseline
  Proteinuria
  More than 300 mg in a 24-hour period

  Urine protein concentration of at least 1 g/L in two random urine specimens collected at least 6 hours apart
  Edema and generalized weight gain of more than 5 lb in a week

  These changes must have occurred after the twentieth week of gestation
- Features of severe pregnancy-induced hypertension:
  Blood pressure greater than 160/110 mm Hg

  More than 5 g proteinuria in a 24-hour period or 3+ or 4+ proteinuria noted on semiquantitative assay

  Oliguria (< 500 ml/day)

  Cerebral or visual disturbances
  Pulmonary edema
  Epigastric or right upper quadrant pain
  Deranged liver functions
  Thrombocytopenia
- Factors predisposing to preeclampsia:
  Occurs in about 5% of pregnancies
  Family history
  Nulliparity
  Diabetes
  Multiple gestation
  Renal disease
  Hydatiform mole
  Poor prenatal care
- Other features of preeclampsia:
  Patient may have falsely high hematocrit because of hypovolemia and hemoconcentration

  HELLP syndrome (hemolysis, elevated liver enzymes, low platelet) seen in 10% of patients with pregnancy-induced hypertension

  DIC uncommon

  PCWP usually low, cardiac index usually normal or low, and elevated mean PAP

  Preeclampsia typically regresses rapidly after delivery

  Low doses of aspirin and dietary calcium supplementation may have some role in the prevention of preeclampsia
- Eclampsia is the presence of seizures in addition to preeclampsia criteria. It occurs in about 1 in 700 pregnancies. The seizures may occur before, during, or after delivery. Postpartum eclampsia almost always occurs within 24 hours of delivery. Any seizure activity developing more than 48 hours postpartum merits further investigation.

MANAGEMENT OF PREECLAMPSIA AND ECLAMPSIA

- Hospitalize patient if you suspect preeclampsia
- *Fluid therapy*: cautious volume expansion with crystalloid or small volumes of high molecular weight solutions
- Preventing and controlling convulsions

   The data from the recently published Collaborative Eclampsia Trial have clearly demonstrated that magnesium sulphate is superior to both diazepam and phenytoin in preventing recurrent seizures. Furthermore, both maternal and fetal outcome was better in those patients who received magnesium sulphate

   Intravenous and intramuscular magnesium sulfate dosing regimen: intravenous loading with 4 to 6 g of 20% solution at 1 g/min and a maintenance dose of 5 g of 50% solution IM every 4 hr. Continue magnesium sulfate for 24 hours after all seizures have stopped

   Intravenous magnesium sulfate dosing regimen: 6 g loading dose at 1 g/min, followed by 2 g/hr maintenance dose

   Aim for target serum level of 4 to 6 mEq/L. Monitor urine output, deep patellar reflex, and respiratory status. If patient develops respiratory depression, you may give 1 g of 10% calcium gluconate solution as an antidote. If the patient develops respiratory failure, intubation and mechanical ventilation may be required

   Parenterally administered magnesium is cleared almost totally by renal excretion. In patients with renal impairment, the dosage must be adjusted according to calculated creatinine clearance

   Patients may need additional magnesium sulfate (2 g of 20% solution intravenously) if seizures are not controlled. If still uncontrolled, you may give 250 mg sodium amobarbital and monitor oxygenation and ventilation

Maintain airway, prevent tongue laceration, place patient in left lateral position to decrease aspiration risk and maintain blood return from IVC

- Control of blood pressure (also see Chapter 17)

  The goal is to keep BP in the 140 to 150/90 to 100 range

  5 to 10 mg hydralazine intravenously every 20 minutes

  May use labetalol or nifedipine if BP is still uncontrolled

  Nicardipine (dihydropyridine calcium channel blocker) has recently been released in an intravenous form and may prove useful in this disorder

  Avoid ACE inhibitors. Use is associated with fetal death and hypotension in neonate

  Avoid diuretics since they further compromise placental perfusion by reducing an already decreased intravascular volume

  In severe cases sodium nitroprusside may be used (fetus at risk for cyanide toxicity)

  Nitroglycerin and diuretics may be needed for associated pulmonary edema

- Indications for pulmonary artery catheterization

  Pulmonary edema or ARDS

  Oliguria, unresponsive to initial volume expansion

  Severe hypertension unresponsive to vasodilator therapy

  Maternal cardiac disease

  Shock

- Initiating delivery

An expectant approach aimed at prolonging pregnancy is associated with high maternal morbidity and high perinatal mortality. Prompt delivery is indicated if the patient is near term, has severe hypertension persisting after 24 to 48 hours of treatment, low platelet count, liver or renal dysfunction, or if premonitory signs of eclampsia (headache, hyperreflexia) are present.

Vaginal delivery is preferred, with amniotomy and induction of labor.

Perform a cesarean delivery in event of fetal compromise.

AMNIOTIC FLUID EMBOLISM

- Characterized by a state of profound shock, developing suddenly and unexpectedly, during or shortly after delivery. It occurs as a result of embolization of amniotic fluid containing squamous cells, meconium, mucin, lanugo hair, and fat into maternal circulation
- Exact incidence not know, probably 1 in 8000 to 80,000 live births
- Very high maternal mortality (80% to 90%)
- Can be associated with abortion, amniocentesis, uncomplicated pregnancy, placental abruption, cesarean section, intrauterine death, violent labor, multiparity, and macrosomic fetus
- Presents as abrupt cardiopulmonary collapse (hypotension and hypoxia) without a significant prodrome. Later pulmonary edema develops as a result of left ventricular failure. Bronchospasm is unusual. About 10% to 15% of patients may also develop seizures or DIC along with collapse.
- The manifestations of amniotic fluid embolism are probably the result of a mechanical obstruction of

the pulmonary vasculature, alveolar capillary leak leading to ARDS, left ventricular dysfunction, and anaphylactic reaction to fetal antigens.

- The diagnosis is difficult. One needs a high suspicion in the right setting.
- *Pulmonary microvascular cytology (PMVC)*: blood sample from distal port of PA catheter in wedged position may show a large number of fetal squames (flat, polygonal, keratinized, anucleate cells), mucin, and hair. PMVC showing squames with mucin and hair or squames coated with neutrophils strongly support the diagnosis of amniotic fluid embolism.
- Management is supportive. Most patients will need intubation and mechanical ventilation with PEEP. A PA catheter is needed for hemodynamic monitoring and PMVC. Hypotension should be corrected. Avoid fluid overloading. Replacement therapy with packed red cells and FFP is indicated in the event of severe coagulopathy and hemorrhage. There is no role for anticoagulants, corticosteriods, or empiric antibiotics in this disorder.

TOCOLYTIC-INDUCED PULMONARY EDEMA

- Beta-adrenergic agents (ritodrine, terbutaline, isoxsuprine) are widely used for inhibition of preterm labor.
- Maternal pulmonary edema is seen in 4% to 5% of such cases
- Pathophysiology is not clear since both normal and high filling pressures have been seen on PA monitoring.
- Typically, patients develop chest discomfort, dyspnea, chest pain, cough, tachypnea, crackles, and evidence of pulmonary edema on chest radiograph within 48 hours of starting tocolytic therapy.
- Hypotension and clotting abnormalities are uncommon.
- Discontinue tocolytic therapy at the first symptoms suggestive of pulmonary edema. Mechanical ventila-

tion is rarely needed. Rarely, diuretics and PA catheterization may be required. Immediate delivery is not
mandatory. First stablilize the patient, and then
deliver the fetus.

- It can be prevented by proper patient selection.
Avoid tocolytics in patients with preeclampsia, thyrotoxicosis, hypervolemia, and severe asthmatics on
beta-agonists. Also avoid using tocolytics for more
than 24 to 48 hours.

ABRUPTIO PLACENTAE

- Incidence of about 1 in 120 deliveries
- Cause is unknown but is associated with hypertensive disorders, parity, previous abruption, cocaine
abuse, and trauma
- The patient presents with abdominal pain, which
may be associated with vaginal bleeding
- Fetal condition depends on the duration and degree
of separation of the placenta
- Management:
- Establish adequate venous access, crossmatch blood,
order coagulation studies
- Monitor maternal hemodynamics and fetal heart rate
- The decision to allow vaginal delivery or to proceed
with cesaerean section (if the fetus is alive) are
dependent on the condition of both the mother and
the fetus

ACUTE FATTY LIVER OF PREGNANCY

- Acute hepatic dysfunction that develops late in pregnancy and is associated with microvesicular fat accumulation in hepatocyte
- More common with twin pregnancies and is associated with preeclampsia in up to half of the cases
- Occurs typically after the thirtieth week of gestation

- Present as nausea, vomiting, malaise, abdominal pain, and then hepatic failure, jaundice, encephalopathy
- Incidence of 1 in 13,000 deliveries, fetal mortality 23%, maternal mortality 18%
- Death usually occurs because of sepsis, hemorrhage, or hypoglycemia
- Therapy is mainly supportive. Monitor for and treat bleeding, sepsis, and hypoglycemia. Immediate delivery is probably beneficial since there are no reports of recovery before delivery

PERIPARTUM CARDIOMYOPATHY

- Patients present in the last month of pregnancy or the first 6 months after delivery (most patients present in the first 3 months postpartum). By definition the patient has no preexisting heart disease, and there are no other identifiable causes of heart failure
- It is seen in 1 in 3000 to 4000 deliveries. It is more common among black women, multiple gestation, toxemia, and the presence of postpartum hypertension.
- Patients typically present with features of congestive heart failure (elevated JVD, S_3 gallop, cardiomegaly, edema, mitral regurgitation murmur). Chest radiograph demonstrates cardiomegaly and pulmonary edema and occasionally pleural effusions. Echocardiography will show global hypokinesia.
- Peripartum cardiomyopathy is a diagnosis of exclusion. Congenital and valvular heart disease and metabolic and toxic disorders causing heart failure must be excluded.
- Therapy involves the use of digoxin and diuretics. ACE inhibitors should be used in postpartum patients. Patients with intractable heart failure are candidates for cardiac transplantation. Systemic anticoagulation is indicated because of the high risk of systemic and pulmonary emboli in these patients.

Cases with severe decompensation occurring in the third trimester may require PA catheter monitoring during labor and delivery.

- These patients have high mortality—up to 50% dying in the first 3 months postpartum. In survivors, it tends to recur in subsequent pregnancies especially if heart size does not return to normal size in 6 to 12 months after initial episode.

CHAPTER 60

Routine chest radiograph

A number of studies have demonstrated that routine daily chest radiographic examinations in ICU patients frequently demonstrate new, unexpected, or changing abnormalities, which result in changes in therapy. Daily portable chest examinations should therefore be performed in all but the most stable ICU patients. Daily chest radiographs should be performed in all intubated patients.

Interpretation of a bedside film is fraught by numerous pitfalls. All films are AP (anteroposterior) rather than PA (posteroanterior), resulting in magnification of the cardiac silhouette, making interpretation of the cardiothoracic ratio unreliable. Signs of pulmonary venous hypertension (upper lobe vessel recruitment) are difficult to interpret on a supine film. The classic signs of a pneumothorax are not present on the supine chest radiograph. Furthermore, assessment of lung volumes and alveolar infiltrates may be difficult since the films are often of poor quality, taken after a poor inspiratory effort and/or with the patient poorly positioned on the radiographic plate. Notwithstanding these limitations, the routine portable chest radiograph provides vital information that is essential for the management of the critically ill ICU patient.

The chest radiograph should be studied systematically; firstly, the position of all the tubes and catheters should be evaluated, followed by an evaluation of the lung parenchyma, pleura, mediastinum, and diaphragm, followed by a search for signs of extraalveolar air.

POSITION OF TUBES AND CATHETERS

- *Endotracheal tube*: with the patient's head in a neutral position, the tip of the tube should be 7 ± 2 cm from the carina. It should be noted that with movement of the head, from a flexed to to an extended position, the tube can move by as much as 4 cm. A useful landmark for the tip of the ET tube is the superior border of the aortic notch (Lipman sign) or the upper border of T4.
- *Central venous catheters*: the tip of the catheter should be located beyond the venous valves of the subclavian or internal jugular vein but proximal to the right atrium (i.e., above the superior vena cava-right atrial junction). Placement in the right atrium may result in atrial perforation. The following are two useful radiographic landmarks for the position of the tip of the catheter:

    The first costochondral junction
    A point 2 cm inferior to a line joining inferior margins of the clavicular heads
- *Pulmonary artery catheter*: the tip of the pulmonary artery catheter should be located in the proximal left or right branch of the pulmonary artery.
- *The position of other tubes and catheters, such as the nasogastric tube, feeding tube, chest tubes, intraaortic balloon catheter and pacing wires should be noted.*

LUNG PARENCHYMA, PLEURA, AND MEDIASTINUM

- *Pulmonary infiltrates*: the presence of pulmonary infiltrates should be noted. It should be noted whether the infiltrate is interstitial or alveolar (or both), unilateral or bilateral, and patchy or diffuse. An infiltrate may be caused by either *water* (cardiogenic or noncardiogenic pulmonary edema), *cells* (infection), and/or *blood* (pulmonary hematoma, intraalveolar bleeding). It should be appreciated that it may not be possible to distinguish among these entities by examination of the chest film alone. The following radiographic findings may help distinguish cardiac and noncardiac pulmonary edema:

Noncardiac pulmonary edema (acute lung injury)
  Normal heart shape
  Absence of septal lines
  No peribronchial cuffing
  Frequent air bronchograms
  Patchy increased lung density
  Peripheral increased lung density
Cardiogenic pulmonary edema
  Base-to-apex blood flow inversion
  Even distribution of increased lung density
  Septal lines
  Peribronchial cuffing

Lipman's rule: the only infiltrate that clears radiographically within 24 hours is fluid (pulmonary edema).

- *Pleural fluid*: in the supine position fluid tracks posteriorly, resulting in a diffuse haziness of the lung fields. It is therefore very easy to miss a significant pleural collection. Fluid collections can be confirmed by lateral decubitus films or ultrasonography.
- *The width of the mediastinum should be noted* (normal; < 10 cm) as well as the presence of mediastinal nodes or masses.
- *Evidence of barotrauma*: the traditional apicolateral collection of air may not be present on portable supine films of patients with pneumothoraces. Free air will often be located in the anterior costophrenic sulcus, since this is the most superior portion of the pleural space in the supine patient. Other radiographic signs of a pneumothorax in the supine position include a relative hyperlucency over the upper abdominal quadrants and a deep costophrenic angle (the deep sulcus sign).

CHAPTER 61

Drug monitoring in the ICU

Refer to Table 61-1. The timing of the serum specimen for drug analysis is important. With intermittent dosing, a steady state is achieved after approximately 4 to 5 half-lives (beta half-life). A steady state is achieved much sooner in patients who have received a loading dose of the drug. Furthermore, after administration of an oral or IV dose, it takes time for the drug to equilibrate with the extravascular compartment (alpha half-life). A specimen taken during this equilibration time will give erroneously high results.

Aminoglycoside and vancomycin peak levels should be taken 1 hour after the end of the infusion. Trough levels should be taken just before the next dose. Digoxin levels should be taken 6 hours after the last IV dose and 12 hours after the last oral dose. Phenobarbital, phenytoin, and carbamazepine should be taken at steady state before the next dose. Serum levels of drugs given as a constant infusion (after a loading dose) should be taken 6 hours after the initiation of the infusion (aminophylline, lidocaine, procainamide).

Table 61-1 Drug monitoring in the ICU

Drug	Half-life (hr)	Desired blood levels
Amikacin	2-3	Peak > 30 µg/ml Trough < 5 µg/ml
Gentamicin/ Tobramycin	2-3	Peak 5-10 µg/ml Trough < 2 µg/ml
Vancomycin	6-10	Peak 25-40 µg/ml Trough < 10 µg/ml
Carbamazepine	12-17	4-12 µg/ml
Phenobarbital	75-126	10-30 µg/ml
Phenytoin	10-34	10-20 µg/ml Free 1-2 µg/ml
Valproic acid	6-18	50-100 µg/ml
Theophylline	8-9	10-15 (up to 20) µg/ml
Digoxin	36-48	1-2 ng/ml
Lidocaine	1.5-2	1-5 µg/ml
Quinidine	6-7	1-4 µg/ml
Procainamide	3-4	4-8 µg/ml
Cyclosporine	18-36	100-300 ng/ml

CHAPTER 62

Alcohol intoxication and withdrawal syndrome

Refer to Table 62-1.

MEDICAL COMPLICATIONS ASSOCIATED WITH ACUTE ALCOHOL INGESTION

- Acute myopathy with rhabdomyolysis
- Gastritis
- Esophagitis
- Mallory-Weiss syndrome
- Thrombocytopenia
- Pancreatitis

Table 62-1 Alcohol intoxication

Blood ethanol concentration (mg/dl)	Symptoms
50-150	Euphoria or dysphoria. Uninhibited, impaired concentration, and judgment
150-250	Slurred speech, ataxic gait, drowsiness, labile moods, antisocial behavior
250-400	Stupor, incoherent speech, vomiting
400-500	Coma
> 500	Death

- Alcoholic hepatitis
- Arrhythmias, especially atrial fibrillation
- Decreased myocardial contractility (synergistic with cocaine)
- Peripheral vasodilation and hypotension
- Alcohol withdrawal syndrome and delirium tremens
- Hypoglycemia
- Electrolyte disturbances, including hypokalemia, hyponatremia, hypophosphatemia, hypomagnesemia
- Wernicke syndrome

TREATMENT OF ETHANOL WITHDRAWAL SYNDROME AND DELIRIUM TREMENS

- Benzodiazipines are the drugs of choice for treating alcohol withdrawal syndrome
- All the benzodiazepines are metabolized by the liver (see Table 43-3). There are no data to suggest that one agent is better than another. In general, patients with minor withdrawal can be treated with a long-acting oral agent (chlordiazepoxide or diazepam). An intravenous, intermediate acting agent (lorazepam) is preferred for more serious cases.
- In patients with moderate to severe alcohol withdrawal, it is critically important to rapidly achieve adequate sedation. This is best achieved by using small boluses of lorazepam (1 to 2 mg IV) q 10 to 15 minutes until the patient is adequately sedated. Titrate to effect and *not* total dose. These patients may require very large doses of benzodiazepines.
- Once the patient is adequately sedated, a maintenance dose of a benzodiazepine is required to maintain sedation and anxiolysis. This can be achieved using either with an oral benzodiazepine or intermittent boluses of lorazepam. Patients with severe withdrawal syndrome are best managed with a lorazepam infusion.
- Thiamine 100 mg stat, then thiamine and multivitamins daily

- Phosphate, potassium and magnesium supplementation; check levels
- Hyperadrenergic patients
  Beta-blockade: atenolol 50 qd/bd or metoprolol 100 qd/bd and/or

  Clonidine 0.1 mg PO q 6 to 8 hr or 0.1 to 0.2 mg/day transdermal
- Haloperidol may be useful for controlling delirium.
- Ethanol withdrawal seizures should be treated with diazepam and/or midazolam. Phenytoin has not been shown to reduce the risk of recurrent seizures. A CT scan should always be obtained to exclude a structural cause of seizures (e.g., subdural hematoma).

CHAPTER 63

Medical complications of cocaine abuse

During the last decade, cocaine use has become a major social problem in the United States. An estimated 30 million people have tried cocaine, and some 3 to 5 million individuals abuse it regularly. Cocaine abuse is associated with a wide range of medical complications, many of which may be life threatening, requiring treatment in an ICU.

Cocaine is an alkaloid derived from the coca plant, which is native to South America. Cocaine hydrochloride is a water-soluble powder that can be absorbed through the nasal mucosa or injected intravenously. Cocaine hydrochloride has a high melting point and decomposes when burnt; this form of cocaine is therefore not suitable for smoking. Cocaine can be effectively smoked when it has been transformed into an alkaloid form, either "freebase" or "crack." Freebase and crack are the same chemical form of cocaine but are made using different techniques.

PHARMACODYNAMICS AND PHARMACOKINETICS

Cocaine acts by blocking the reuptake of neurotransmitters (norepinephrine, dopamine, and serotonin) at synaptic junctions, resulting in increased neurotransmitter concentrations. This results in sympathic and central nervous stimulation.

Cocaine can be smoked, nasally insufflated, or injected intravenously. Smoking "crack" cocaine is a popular and potentially dangerous route of administration. Because of the large absorptive surface area of the lung, very high serum levels can be achieved within seconds. Nasal insufflation produces euphoria in about 3 to 5 minutes, with peak cocaine levels being achieved in 30 to 60 minutes. The biologic half-life in the blood is about 1 hour. Cocaine is metabolized to benzoylecgonine and ecgonine, which are excreted in the urine. Less than 5% of cocaine is excrete unchanged in the urine. Most urinary excretion occurs within 24 hours of administration. Most assays for detecting cocaine measure urinary benzoylecgonine levels. This assay will be positive for up to 6 days after a single use and as long as 21 days with high dose, long-term use.

ALCOHOL AND COCAINE: A DEADLY COMBINATION

Alcohol enhances the euphoric effects of cocaine, and approximately 12 million Americans use this drug combination. *Cocaethylene* is produced by the liver from the combination of cocaine and ethanol. Cocaethylene produces intense dopaminergic stimulation in the brain and myocardium. The risk of sudden death is 25 times greater in persons who abuse both alcohol and cocaine than in those who use only cocaine.

MEDICAL COMPLICATIONS

- *Sudden death* is caused by arrhythmias, intracerebral bleeds, respiratory arrest

  BOOP (bronchiolitis obliterans with organizing pneumonia)

  Pneumothorax and pneumomediastinum
  Interstitial pneumonitis

- Neurological
  Seizures
  Hemorrhagic strokes
  Cerebral infarctions
  Ruptured aneurysms
- Renal
  Rhabdomyolysis and acute renal failure
- Other
  Intestinal ischemia
  Gastroduodenal perforations
  DIC
  Placental abruption
  Hyperthermia

THE MANAGEMENT OF COCAINE TOXICITY

- Agitation is best treated with benzodiazepines
- *Seizures*: solitary seizures usually do not require therapy. Status epilepticus, however, requires aggressive treatment with intravenous benzodiazepines followed by a loading dose of phenytoin.
- Hyperthermia must be treated immediately with cool-water washes and/or with cooling blankets.
- *Hypertension*: this is usually self-limiting. However, severe or sustained hypertension should be treated with labetalol, nitroprusside, or nicardipine. *Beta-blockers may cause paradoxical worsening of hypertension as a result of unopposed alpha stimulation.*
- *Myocardial infarction*: administration of thrombolytic agents remains controversial. In cases of myocardial ischemia or impending infarction, calcium channel blockers, aspirin, and nitroglycerin are recommended. Patients with hyperadrenergic signs may benefit from labetalol (see above).
- *Detoxification*: the combination of bromocriptine and desipramine is currently recommended.

CHAPTER 64

Toxicology

GENERAL MEASURES

- Stabilization of patient, i.e., airway, breathing, and circulation

    Intubate obtunded and comatose patients and seizing patient

    Obtain IV access

    Treat hypotension initially with volume expansion
- Comatose patients should be given naloxone 0.8 mg IV
- Flumazenil (a benzodiazepine antagonist) may be indicated for patients who present with obtundation or coma. An initial dose of 0.2 mg intravenously should be given over 30 seconds. Additional doses of 0.2 to 0.5 mg can be given for up to a total of 3 mg
- *Ipecac is not recommended for most ingestions*
- Gastric lavage is indicated in the following circumstances:

    Recent ingestion (< 1 hour) of a potentially life-threatening poison

    Ingestion of a substance that slows gastric emptying (e.g., anticholinergic medications)

    Ingestion of a poison that is slowly absorbed from the gastrointestinal tract

    Ingestion of a substance that does not bind well to activated charcoal (see p. 384)

Ingestion of specific life-threatening poisons (e.g., tricyclic antidepressants, theophylline, cyanide)
- Technique for performing gastric lavage

Patients who cannot protect their airway *must be intubated* before gastric lavage is performed

Patient should be placed in head down lateral position

Place large-bore lavage tube through mouth
Aspirate to empty stomach

Lavage with 150 to 300 ml tepid tap water
Contraindicated in caustic ingestions
- *Activated charcoal*: this is the *cornerstone of most ingestions*. Activated charcoal is administered in a dose of 50 to 100 g.

The following are drugs that are not well bound to activated charcoal:
  Bromides
  Caustics
  Cyanide
  Ethylene glycol
  Heavy metals
  Iron
  Isopropyl alcohol
  Lithium
  Methanol

The following are drugs amenable to repeat-dose activated charcoal therapy:
  Carbamazepine
  Nadolol
  Phenobarbital
  Procainamide
  Quinidine
  Sotalol
  Thallium
  Ethanol
  Methanol
  Ethylene glycol

Isopropanol
Aspirin
Lithium
Bromide
Arsenic

Refer to Table 64-1.

CARBON MONOXIDE POISONING AND SMOKE INHALATION

See Chapter 56.

Table 64-1 Toxic substances with specific antidotes

Agent	Antidote
Acetaminophen	N-acetylcysteine
Anticholinergic poisoning	Physostigmine
Anticoagulants	Vitamin K, protamine
Benzodiazepines	Flumazenil
Beta-adrenergic antagonists	Glucagon, calcium salts, isoproterenol
Carbon monoxide	Oxygen, hyperbaric oxygen
Cholinergic syndrome	Atropine
Digoxin	Fab Antibody, Mg
Ethylene glycol	Ethanol, thiamine
Fluoride	Calcium and Mg salts
Heavy metals	BAL, DMSA, D-penicillamine
Iron	Deferoxamine
Isoniazid	GABA agonists, pyridoxine
Methemoglobinemia	Methylene blue
Opoids	Naloxone

SPECIFIC INTOXICATIONS

Acetaminophen

- Signs and symptoms

  Stage 1: 12 to 24 hours after ingestion; asymptomatic or mild GI symptoms

  Stage 2: 24-72 hours; disappearance of symptoms, liver enzymes begin to rise.

  Stage 3: 72-96 hours; patient either improves with normalization of enzymes or progresses to acute hepatic necrosis with liver failure

- Management

  Analyzing the serum acetaminophen concentration is essential in all cases of overdose. A level taken before 4 hours is difficult to interpret. High potential for toxicity exists when serum concentration is > 200 µg/ml at 4 hours, 50 µg/ml at 12 hours, and 7 µg/ml at 24 hours after ingestion.

  N-acetylcysteine should be administered as soon as possible within the first 24 hours of ingestion. However, antidotal therapy is optimal when given within 12 hours of acetaminophen ingestion. *N*-acetylcysteine should be given if the patient has ingested more than 140 mg/kg (or 10 g) acetaminophen, if the serum level is above 140 µg/ml, or if the serum level is in the toxic range (Fig. 64-1). The dose of *N*-acetylcysteine is 140 mg/kg as an initial oral loading dose, followed by 70 mg/kg every 4 hours for a total of 17 doses.

- It may be useful to measure a second level some time after starting *N*-acetylcysteine to determine the half-life of acetaminophen. A half-life greater than 4 hours is suggestive of hepatic toxicity. *N*-acetylcysteine should not be stopped as the level falls to zero, since it is not acetaminophen that is toxic but rather its metabolites.

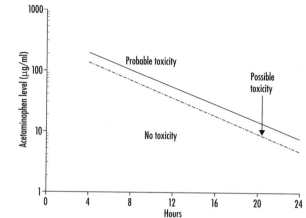

Fig. 64-1 Acetaminophen nomogram.

Antidepressants

- Signs and symptoms

  Anticholinergic: mydriasis, blurred vision, dry mouth, tachycardia, hyperpyrexia, urinary retention, decreased GI motility

  CNS: agitation, mental confusion, respiratory depression, seizures, coma

  Cardiac: quinidine-like action on heart; widened QRS, PR, and QT intervals; RBBB; torsades de pointe. The best predictor of cardiac arrhythmias and seizures is a QRS complex greater than 0.1 seconds or a prolonged QTc interval.

- Management

  Antidepressants are highly tissue bound, and therefore serum concentrations do not correlate with toxicity and have little clinical value.

  Supportive measures: GI decontamination and activated charcoal are essential.

- Alkalinization of the serum with bicarbonate to achieve an arterial pH of 7.5 to 7.55 should be instituted in patients with a prolonged QRS/QTc interval or cardiac arrhythmias. Alkalinization increases plasma protein binding (less free drug) and antagonizes the quinidine-like effects on the His-Purkinje system.
- Seizures are best treated with diazepam and midazolam or intravenous phenobarbital. Phenytoin is ineffective and may be dangerous
- Lidocaine should be used for ventricular arrhythmias. Phenytoin improves conduction through the specialized conduction tissue of the heart and is considered by some to be the drug of choice in this setting. Since 20 to 30 minutes is required to deliver a 15 mg/kg loading dose of phenytoin, bicarbonate and lidocaine should be used as initial therapy to control ventricular arrhythmias.

Refer to Table 64-2.

THEOPHYLLINE

- Signs and symptoms
    Nausea, vomiting, diarrhea, abdominal pain, tremors, headache, cardiac arrhythmias, hypotension, seizures, coma, death
- Management
    Gastric lavage
    Activated charcoal
    Monitor blood levels
    Correct potassium, calcium, and magnesium
    Charcoal hemoperfusion:
        Acute exposure
            Age < 60 years plasma level > 100 μg/ml
            Age > 60 years plasma level > 40 to 50 μg/ml
        Chronic exposure
            Age < 60 years plasma level > 60 μg/ml
            Age > 60 years plasma level > 30 to 40 μg/ml
        Any life-threatening poisoning regardless of level

Table 64-2 Antidepressant drugs

Antidepressent	Sedative	Orthostatic	Anticholinergic	Conduction disturbance or arrhythmia	Daily dosage range (mg)
Tricyclic					
Doxepin	High	Moderate	Moderate	Yes	25–400
Amitriptyline	High	Moderate	Highest	Yes	25–300
Imipramine	Moderate	High	Moderate	Yes	50–400
Trimipramine	High	Moderate	Moderate	Yes	50–300
Clomipramine	Moderate	High	High	Yes	75–300
Protriptyline	Lowest	Low	High	Yes	5–60
Nortriptyline	Moderate	Lowest	Moderate	Yes	25–150
Desipramine	Lowest	Low	Moderate	Yes	75–300
Other					
Amoxapine	Moderate	Low	Moderate	Very low	50–300
Maprotiline	Moderate	Low	Moderate	Very low	50–200
Trazodone	Moderate	Moderate	Very low	Very low	50–600
Fluoxetine	Low	Lowest	Low	Low	10–80
Sertraline	Low	Lowest	Low	Low	50–200
Paroxetine	Low	Lowest	Low	Low	10–20
Bupropion	Low	Lowest	Low	Low	75–300

For patients older than 60 years or patients with a history of respiratory failure, congestive heart failure, or liver disease, a theophylline concentration above 40 μg/ml warrants consideration of hemoperfusion. A low threshold for hemoperfusion is recommended for patients taking theophylline chronically, since serum concentrations are not predictive of onset or severity of symptoms and because these patients have the potential to develop life-threatening complications at low serum concentrations.

- Factors affecting serum theophylline level
    - Drugs lowering theophylline levels
        - Carbamazepine
        - Phenobarbital
    - Drugs raising theophylline levels
        - Quinolone antibiotics
        - Oral contraceptives
        - Erythromycin
        - H_2-antagonists
        - Calcium channel blockers
        - Pheyntoin
        - Propranolol
    - Conditions lowering theophylline levels
        - Cigarette smoking
        - Cystic fibrosis
        - Hyperthyroidism
    - Conditions raising serum theophylline levels
        - Hepatitis or cirrhosis
        - Congestive heart failure
        - Some viral infections

DIGITALIS

- Signs and symptons
    - Nausea; vomiting; diarrhea; fatigue; malaise; headache; confusion; delusions; hallucinations; blurred vision; disorder of green-yellow color perception; visualization of halos around objects and life-

threatening cardiac arrhythmias, including paroxysmal atrial tachycardia (PAT) with 2 to 1 block; junctional tachycardia; varying degrees of heart block; ectopy; ventricular tachycardia; ventricular fibrillation

- Management

  Because of a high degree of tissue binding, serum drug levels do not accurately reflect tissue levels. The diagnosis of toxicity is a clinical diagnosis. The majority of patients who show signs of toxicity have a serum level above 2 ng/ml; however, some patients may exhibit toxicity below this level. Similarly patients may have a level above 2 ng/ml with no signs of toxicity.

  Gastric lavage and activated charcoal (acute ingestion)

  Continuous ECG monitoring; evaluate old ECGs

  Correction of electrolytes; beware that K^+ may increase acutely with digoxin overdose

  Atropine for conduction disturbances

  Phenytoin or lidocaine for arrhythmias of impulse formation

  Temporary pacemakers for arrhythmias that are resistant to atropine

  Digoxin-specific antibodies (digoxin FAB fragment antibodies) for serious arrhythmias and severe toxicity:
  Digoxin FAB (Digibind) dosing

  Use extreme caution if patient is in renal failure
  Serum levels not useful once FAB given

  Dose dependent on body load; each vial contains 40 mg FAB and binds 0.6 mg digoxin

Body load of digoxin = (serum digoxin concentration × 5.6 × weight in kg)/1000. Dose (vials) = body load/0.6

SALICYLATES

- Signs and symptoms

    Gastric upset, tinnitus, increased depth of breathing, headache, seizures, coma, anion gap metabolic acidosis, and respiratory alkalosis

- Management

    Serum salicylate levels are useful in confirming the diagnosis and assessing the severity of the toxicity but are not, however, used in directing therapy

    Supportive measures, GI decontamination, and activated charcoal

    Forced alkaline diuresis (ion trapping and increased elimination), in cases of severe toxicity, dialysis is useful. The decision to dialyze the patient is based on clinical grounds, i.e., seizures, altered level of consciousness. Blood level monitoring is useful to monitor drug elimination

Refer to Fig. 64-2.

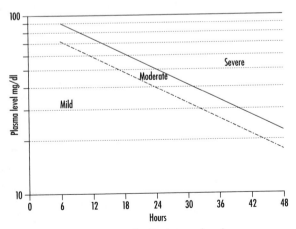

Fig. 64-2 Nomogram of salicylate poisoning.

PHENYTOIN

- Signs and symptoms
  Nystagmus, ataxia, slurred speech, confusion, seizures
- Management
  Phenytoin is highly protein bound, therefore serum levels do not correlate well with toxicity. Free levels are a better indicator of toxicity (< 2 µg/ml). Treatment includes, gastric lavage, and repeated activated charcoal.

PHENCYCLIDINE (PCP)

- Signs and symptoms
  Nystagmus, hypertension, tachycardia, agitation, psychosis, violent behavior and seizures, rhabdomyolysis, and renal failure
- Management
  Test urine for PCP. Check levels of CPK. Supportive measure, benzodiazepines for seizures, vigorous hydration if CPK is elevated

ORGANOPHOSPHATES

- Signs and symptoms
  Muscarinic effects: bronchospasm; bronchorrhea; blurred vision; salivation; lacrimation, urination, defecation (SLUD) syndrome)

  Nicotinic effects: muscle fasciculations, weakness, paralysis, ataxia
- Management
  Decontaminate skin, gastric lavage (ingestion < 1 hour and patient not vomiting) and activated charcoal. An atropine infusion is the mainstay of treatment, the endpoint being the drying of secretions,

particularly bronchial secretions. Pralidoxime 1 to 2 g IV over 15 minutes should be given if the patient seeks treatment within 4 hours of the ingestion.

LITHIUM

- Signs and symptoms

  Mild to moderate toxicity occurs when the serum concentration is between 1.5 and 2.5 mEq/L and severe toxicity when the levels are between 2.5 and 3.5 mEq/L. Levels above 3.5 mEq/L are life threatening. Symptoms, however, do not necessarily correlate with lithium levels, and symptoms of toxicity may occur at therapeutic levels. Neurologic symptoms dominate the clinical picture of lithium toxicity. Symptoms include nausea, vomiting, diarrhea, polyuria, blurred vision, muscular weakness, confusion, vertigo, increased deep tendon reflexes, myoclonus, choreoathetoid movements, urinary and fecal incontinence, stupor, coma, seizures, cardiac arrhythmia, cardiovascular collapse, and death.

- The following are predisposing factors to lithium toxicity:

  Infections
  Volume depletion
  Gastroenteritis
  Renal insufficiency
  Congestive cardiac failure
  Nonsteroidal antiinflammatory drugs
  Diuretics
  Tetracycline

- Management

  Gastric lavage and supportive therapy; activated charcoal is not effective in removing lithium. Dehydrated patients should be actively rehydrated. However, forced saline diuresis is not recommended. Hemodialysis is indicated with levels above 4 mEq/L or in patients with signs of serious toxicity and levels above 2 mEq/L. The duration of dialysis should be guided by the serum levels. It is important to bear in mind that serum levels may rebound up following dialysis and repeat dialysis may be required.

OPIATES

- Signs and symptoms

  Constricted pupils, bradycardia, hypotension, hypothermia, pulmonary edema, respiratory depression, and coma.

- Management

  Management of opiate toxicity includes supportive therapy and the administration of the opiate antagonist naloxone (Narcan). Naloxone should be given as an initial intravenous bolus of 0.4 mg. A bolus of 0.4 mg up to 2 mg can be repeated every 3 to 5 minutes up to a total dose of 10 mg. Naloxone has a duration of action of about 45 to 60 minutes, which is considerably shorter than that of all the opiate agonists. Therefore, should the patient respond to the boluses of naloxone, a continuous infusion should be started, by placing 8 mg into 1000 ml D_5W and infusing at a rate of 0.4 to 0.8 mg/h.

METHANOL AND ETHYLENE GLYCOL POISONING

- Signs and symptoms

  Methanol is metabolized to formaldehyde and formic acid, which are highly toxic metabolites that interfere with mitochondrial respiration and are directly oculotoxic. Features of toxicity include blurred vision, scintillations, loss of sight, unreactive pupils, papilledema, vomiting, epigastric pain, convulsions, coma. Anion gap metabolic acidosis (formate anions).

Ethylene glycol is metabolized to several aldehydes, carboxylic acids, and oxalic acid. These intermediates inhibit cellular respiration, protein synthesis, and RNA replication. Oxalic acid may crystallize as calcium oxalate in many tissues, causing hypocalcemia and tubular obstruction in the kidney. Features of toxicity include confusion, lethargy, coma, seizures, pulmonary edema, respiratory failure, circulatory shock, and renal failure.

- Treatment of methanol and ethylene glycol poisoning The serum methanol and ethylene glycol levels should be measured. However, they can be estimated from the osmolar gap:

$$\text{(Methanol [mg/dl])} = 3.2 \times \text{osmol gap}$$
$$\text{(Ethylene glycol [mg/dl])} = 6.2 \times \text{osmol gap}$$

Syrup of ipecac should be avoided, due to the risk of aspiration. The efficacy of activated charcoal is controversial.

If pH < 7.25, sodium bicarbonate should be given to maintain the pH above 7.25.

Ethanol: ethanol slows down the metabolism of both methanol and ethylene glycol, reducing their toxicity. Ethanol should be given to patients with ocular symptoms (methanol), acidosis, or patients with a serum level greater than 20 mg/dl (methanol and ethylene glycol).

Loading dose: 600 mg/kg IV

Maintenance dose: 100-150 mg/hr. The infusion should be titrated to maintain a serum ethanol level of 100 to 150 mg/dl.

Hemodialysis: hemodialysis facilitates the removal of methanol, ethylene glycol, and their metabolites. Hemodialysis should be instituted in all patients with a serum level above 50 mg/dl, in patients with ocular symptoms (methanol), and in patients with a significant metabolic acidosis. The ethanol infusion rate should be increased during dialysis because it is also removed during dialysis.

Folic and folinic acid: may mitigate the toxic effects of formate, 50 to 100 mg q 4 hr.

ISOPROPYL ALCOHOL

In general isopropyl alcohol is less toxic than either methanol or ethylene glycol. It is metabolized to acetone. Neither a metabolic acidosis nor an ion gap characteristically occur.

- Signs and symptoms

    Dizziness, confusion, slurred speech, headache, ataxia, stupor, and coma

    Nausea, vomiting, abdominal pain, hemorrhagic gastritis, diarrhea

    Hypotension, bradycardia, rhabdomyolysis, hemolysis

- *Management*: treatment is essentially supportive. Hemodialysis is recommended in severe poisoning especially when accompanied by hypotension.

PART EIGHT

IN A LIGHTER VEIN

Murphy's critical care common sense rules

- Don't assume the obvious.
- Uncommon presentations of common diseases are more common than common presentations of uncommon diseases.
- When doing a procedure, remember nature always sides with the hidden flaw. *Corollary:* if something can go wrong it will.
- Just when you think things can't get any worse, they will.
- Never open a can of worms unless you plan to go fishing.
- There are no case reports of patients who have lived forever.
- Good judgment comes from bad experiences. Experience comes from bad judgments.
- *The law of subspecialization:* if you are a hammer, the world looks like a nail.
- An acute surgical abdomen is when a good surgeon says it's an acute surgical abdomen. There is no test for it.
- Before ordering a test, decide what you will do if it is (1) positive or (2) negative. If both answers are the same, don't do the test. *Corollary:* if a test is unlikely to change your management, don't order it.
- If a drug is not working, stop it.
- There is no manifestation that cannot be caused by a given drug.

- Be wary of ex-husbands, ex-wives, and next of kin from far away. They often spell trouble.
- There is no external method to measure the presence or absence of pain.
- It it can't be read, don't write it.
- Avoid the "oliguria-lasix" monosynaptic spinal reflex.
- Listen to the bedside nurse, she or he knows best.
- A surgical patient is but a medical patient with a scar.
- Quality of care is like a good wine—it's impossible to measure but easy to recognize.
- A good clinician knows when to act and when to observe. *Corollary:* doing something harmful is not better than doing nothing.
- The quality of patient care is inversely proportional to the number of consultants on any particular case. *Corollary:* consultitis is a potentially fatal disease.
- Those who can, do; those who cannot, teach. Those who can neither do nor teach, administrate others on how to do and teach.
- A committee is the only life form that has 12 rectums and no brain.
- A simple problem can be made unsolvable if enough committee meetings are held to discuss it.

In conclusion *Confucius* says, "Critical care should be fun. If it's not, it's time to find a new job!"

CHAPTER 66

Murphy's guide to home Swan-Ganz catheter insertion

If you are sick and tired and generally ticked off (DRG: 01011), you need a Swan-Ganz catheter. However, your medical insurance will not pay for the hospital time necessary to place this vital piece of monitoring equipment. Therefore, we have devised the *home insertion kit* for Swan-Ganz catheter placement. Please follow the instructions carefully; failure to do so may lead to death.

- On the morning of surgery, don't eat. Breakfast, including eggs, oatmeal, steak, or coffee is considered eating.
- You will require a mirror, good lighting, and two, perhaps three hands. ECG monitoring is optional.
- Standing in front of the mirror, look at the right side of your neck. If you see a scar from previous carotid surgery, pimples, evidence of radical neck surgery, or massive amounts of hair, look at the left side. If you see the same things, go back to the right, otherwise use the left.
- Use novocaine to deaden the skin, approximately two finger widths above the collar bone and approximately 1 inch lateral to the wind pipe. Good location is critical; if you're not sure, guess (Fig. 66-1).
- Using the long, slightly dull needle, connected to the 10 ml syringe, stick yourself in the spot you anesthetized, aiming at your nipple. Multiple attempts may be necessary. If the needle point comes out of

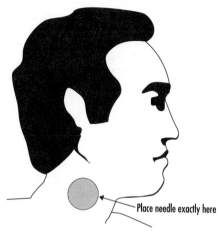

Place needle exactly here

Fig. 66-1 Location for home Swan-Ganz catheter insertion.

your skin, reposition and aim deeper. If you hit a pulsating vessel and the syringe fills with blood, remove the needle and put pressure on the entrance site.

- If, after multiple attempts, you have not found the correct venous structure, try the following:

  Take a deep breath and hold it. This will make the external jugular vein stick out. Still holding your breath, anesthetize the skin over the vein, use the long, dull needle, and advance it until there is a free flow of blood in the syringe. Now, breathe.

- Remove the syringe, and pass the wire through the needle. An occasional extra heart beat confirms proper location. If you seem light-headed or dizzy, you may be in ventricular tachycardia or fibrillation; pull the wire back and hold your breath until you feel better.

- The hard part is over. Remove the needle. Leaving the wire in its place, pass the introducer into the vein. You need not sew it in at this time.

- Place the tip of the Swan into the introducer; advance it to the second mark; pull down the plastic

"condom"; dress the entrance site; and tape the yellow catheter to your forehead. When you get to the hospital, we will do the rest.
- I hope these instructions are clear. If you have any questions, please call your local representative.

Index

B

W